# Rethinking Patient Safety

Kristen Rasmussen

# Rethinking Patient Safety

## Harnessing Design Thinking to Prevent Harm

Springer

Kristen Rasmussen, MSN, RN
Cape Coral, FL, USA

Editorial Contact: Jessica Chio

ISBN 978-3-032-26053-6 ISBN 978-3-032-26054-3 (eBook)
https://doi.org/10.1007/978-3-032-26054-3



This Springer imprint is published by the registered company Springer Nature Switzerland AG
The registered company address is: Gewerbestrasse 11, 6330 Cham, Switzerland

*To all the individuals who care for patients, in every role and at every level: your unwavering and often unseen commitment has shaped my understanding of what safety truly means.*

# Preface

For more than two decades, patient safety has been shaped by investigation. Healthcare professionals have learned to examine adverse events with increasing rigor, evolving and refining root cause analysis, strengthening patient safety reporting systems, and building cultures that acknowledge error rather than conceal it. These efforts have mattered. They have saved lives and transformed how healthcare organizations confront failure. Yet even as safety science has matured, a persistent pattern remains. Many of the same types of events recur. Similar corrective actions reappear. Training is reinforced, policies are revised, compliance improves, and still harm continues.

Over time, a more difficult question began to surface in practice: what if we are not asking the wrong questions about failure, but asking them too late? Working alongside clinicians, quality leaders, human factors specialists, designers, and operational teams, I have witnessed the extraordinary effort required to keep patients safe within complex systems. Much of that effort is adaptive and invisible. People bridge gaps that processes do not anticipate. They work around friction embedded in technology and navigate cognitive load created by misaligned workflows. When harm does not occur, it is often because of human heroics, intervening before system failure. When safety depends on continuous human compensation, the system itself is not inherently reliable. It is sustained by commitment.

This book was written in response to that reality. It does not argue against investigation, accountability, or established safety practices. Retrospective analysis remains essential. Rather, it proposes that investigation alone cannot govern risk in increasingly interdependent healthcare environments. As care becomes more technologically mediated, operationally complex, and socially accountable, safety must move upstream. Anticipation must stand alongside investigation as a core governance function.

Design thinking offers structured methods for doing so. When applied with discipline, it provides ways to observe work as it is performed, surface weak signals before they intensify, test assumptions under realistic conditions, and validate interventions before scale. These methods are not creative exercises detached from safety science. They are mechanisms for strengthening system reliability in environments where variation is inevitable. The aim is pragmatic: to equip healthcare organizations with tools that enable proactive stewardship rather than reactive correction.

Patient safety is not solely a technical discipline. It is also an ethical one. Every preventable injury reflects not only a system breakdown but a misalignment between design and responsibility. If systems are perfectly designed to achieve the results they produce, redesign becomes a professional obligation. The chapters that follow articulate a shift from reactive analysis toward proactive system stewardship, outlining both conceptual foundations and practical methods for integrating design into safety architecture. The intention is to expand the field's capacity to recognize fragility early and to act before harm becomes the catalyst for learning.

Cape Coral, FL, USA Kristen Rasmussen, MSN, RN

# Acknowledgments

I am grateful to the colleagues, mentors, clinicians, operational leaders, quality professionals, and design partners whose insight, candor, and example shaped this work. I am equally grateful to the patients and families whose experiences remain a constant reminder of why patient safety must be pursued with both rigor and humility.

I independently conceived, researched, and wrote this manuscript. A large language model tool was used at a later stage of preparation for limited editorial assistance, including citation formatting review, consistency checks, and minor language refinement. It was not used to generate the book's substantive arguments or original content.

**Competing Interests** The author declares that there are no competing financial or non-financial interests related to the content of this book.

**Ethics Approval** This book does not report primary research involving human participants or animals.

# Contents

# About the Author

**Kristen Rasmussen** MSN, RN, is the Manager of the Innovation Program at Lee Health, where she leads enterprise efforts to integrate human-centered design, strategic transformation, and clinical excellence across acute, ambulatory, and post-acute settings. A nurse leader by training, she previously founded and directed Lee Health's first enterprise Patient Safety Division, aligning multi-setting safety strategy, human factors principles, and executive governance to advance system reliability.

Her work connects frontline clinical insight with organizational design. She has facilitated innovation incubators, design sprints, and cross-functional strategy initiatives focused on workforce models, virtual care, care delivery redesign, and health system transformation. She has completed formal training in user experience design and change management, strengthening her ability to translate systems thinking into practical, scalable implementation within complex healthcare environments.

Kristen holds a Master of Science in Nursing Leadership from Walden University and a Bachelor of Science in Nursing from Drexel University. She has presented nationally on patient safety and innovation. *Beyond Root Cause Analysis: Design Thinking for Proactive Patient Safety* reflects her devotion to advancing anticipatory governance and strengthening reliability in modern healthcare systems.

# A New Era of Patient Safety

# 1

## Introduction

Patient safety has remained a central concern in healthcare policy and practice since the late twentieth century. More than two decades have passed since the Institute of Medicine's landmark report *To Err Is Human* estimated that somewhere between 44,000 and 98,000 patients die each year in U.S. hospitals due to preventable medical errors [1]. Subsequent studies have revised these figures upward, with some estimates suggesting that over 200,000 Americans die annually because of healthcare-associated harm, placing medical error among the leading causes of death in the United States [2, 3].

The scale of the problem is not confined to the United States. The World Health Organization reports that adverse events due to unsafe care rank among the ten leading causes of death and disability worldwide. At least one in ten patients is harmed while receiving hospital care in high-income countries, and rates are often higher in low-resource settings [4]. The effects of harm are not limited to physical injury. Patients and families may experience psychological trauma, loss of trust, and lasting uncertainty. Healthcare professionals may carry moral distress, guilt, and exhaustion long after the formal review of an event has concluded. These effects are often compounded by opaque accountability structures, inconsistent organizational learning, and cultures that privilege compliance more readily than reflection [5].



K. Rasmussen, *Rethinking Patient Safety*,
https://doi.org/10.1007/978-3-032-26054-3_1

Despite substantial focus and investment in quality improvement (QI) initiatives, clinical governance structures, and safety-related technologies, including computerized physician order entry, barcoded medication administration, and electronic health records, progress has remained uneven [6]. In some cases, technologies introduced in the name of safety have generated new risks of their own, contributing to what has been described as e-iatrogenesis: harm arising from health information technology rather than from the clinical treatment it is meant to support [7].

Why does preventable harm remain so persistent in a field that has studied it so closely? Traditional safety science has emphasized linear causality, safety event reporting, and root cause analysis (RCA), often grounded in assumptions drawn from industrial and aviation models of error prevention [8]. While these frameworks have been instrumental in highlighting system-level vulnerabilities, they are increasingly critiqued for their limited adaptability to the dynamic, interdependent realities of clinical care [9].

This chapter proceeds from a different starting point. It treats harm not simply as an anomalous breakdown within an otherwise sound system but as evidence that the system may not be well fitted to the work it requires people to do. When clinicians create work-arounds, when patients disengage from plans of care, or when teams compensate repeatedly for awkward processes and poorly aligned technologies, these conditions warrant more than behavioral correction. They warrant examination of the design of the system itself. Such examination includes attention to workflow fit, cognitive demand, communication burden, environmental constraint, and the broader sociotechnical conditions within which care is delivered.

Meaningful improvement therefore requires more than expanded compliance and more refined counting of events. It requires closer examination of how care is actually delivered, how strain accumulates in everyday work, and how system design shapes both failure and successful recovery. Human-centered design, human factors engineering, and user experience design offer methods for pursuing this work [10–12]. These approaches have already informed redesign efforts in intensive care settings [13], digital health access [10], and maternal safety infrastructure [14].

The chapter begins by examining why traditional safety models plateau. It then considers harm as a system signal, introduces design thinking as a methodology for patient safety, and concludes by addressing the organizational and leadership implications of this change.

## Why Traditional Safety Models Plateau

Patient safety strategies have long emphasized error prevention through standardized processes and post-event analysis. These approaches have improved consistency, clarified accountability, and strengthened institutional attention to harm. Their limitations become more visible, however, in environments where care is variable, distributed, time-sensitive, and dependent on ongoing adaptation.

### The Safety Paradigm: Avoiding Error, Missing Insight

Root cause analysis (RCA) remains one of the most familiar tools in patient safety. Its purpose is to trace an adverse event back to a single, identifiable "root cause" and prescribe corrective actions to prevent recurrence. RCA can be useful in clarifying process breakdowns and organizing the immediate narrative of an event. Its limitations become more evident when the event in question has not arisen from a single upstream cause, but from multiple interacting conditions that shift over time [8].

Healthcare rarely behaves as a simple chain of cause and effect. Adverse events frequently emerge from complex interactions among people, technologies, environments, and institutional expectations [15]. Yet RCA often encourages a level of explanatory closure that does not fully match those conditions. Recommendations then follow a familiar pattern: additional training, another reminder, stricter adherence to policy, or reinforcement of existing procedure. These responses are often easy to issue and easy to document, but they are less effective when the underlying problem lies in system fit rather than in awareness alone.

Empirical studies of RCA in healthcare have shown that similar categories of events recur across settings despite repeated investigation and intervention, including medication errors, communication failures, and equipment misuse [16, 17]. This does not render RCA obsolete. It does, however, suggest that retrospective explanation is insufficient when the same underlying pressures continue to generate the same forms of breakdown.

This orientation reflects what Hollnagel terms Safety-I: a framework in which safety is defined largely as the absence of adverse outcomes and improvement is pursued through reduction of deviation, increased standardization, and tighter control [9]. Safety-I has shaped a substantial portion of modern patient safety work. Its contribution has been significant. Its limitations are now also clearer. In particular, it tends to position human variability primarily as a hazard to be constrained rather than as a condition through which safety is often actively maintained.

Most care is delivered without incident, not because the surrounding systems are perfectly designed, but because clinicians continuously adjust. They reprioritize tasks, recover from interruptions, clarify ambiguity, bridge weak handoffs, and adapt to the demands of the moment. These adjustments are not incidental to safety. In many cases, they are among the principal means through which safety is produced in practice [9, 18].

## Mind the Stakeholder Gap

A further limitation of traditional safety approaches lies in the distance between those who define problems and those who experience them directly. Safety strategies are frequently shaped by leaders, regulators, or quality authorities, while patients, families, nurses, pharmacists, and other frontline staff enter the process later, or only after harm has occurred [19]. Even when frontline perspectives are invited in, they are often limited to retrospective review rather than incorporated into early problem definition or solution design.

This gap matters because an intervention can appear entirely reasonable at the level of policy and still function poorly in real use. A process that fits one clinical area may become cumbersome, misaligned, or unsafe in another. Staffing patterns vary. Physical environments differ. Patient populations differ. Tools that function well under one set of conditions may create a burden or confusion under another [20].

Standardization remains an important part of patient safety work. Problems arise when standardization is treated as sufficient in itself, without close attention to context, usability, and the realities of everyday clinical work. Under those conditions, organizations may achieve visible compliance without producing more reliable care.

## A Shift Towards Resilience and Adaptation

In response to these limitations, safety scholars have advanced what is often described as Safety-II. Rather than concentrating exclusively on failure, Safety-II examines how care succeeds under variable conditions [18]. This move expands the field of inquiry. It asks how safe performance is sustained, what kinds of adaptation are routinely required, and what those adaptations reveal about the system in which they occur.

From this perspective, many failures begin as mismatches. The issue may lie in a tool that does not fit the task, a communication platform that fragments information, a workflow that adds burden at precisely the wrong point, or an organizational expectation that assumes more time, attention, or coordination than the setting can support. In such cases, harm is not well understood as the breakdown of an otherwise well-functioning machine. It is more accurately understood as a sign that the system has been depending on compensation for some time.

## Reframing Harm: From Event to System Signal

Traditional safety reviews often begin with the event itself: the missed dose, the delayed diagnosis, the failed handoff. If this type of approach is asking, "What went wrong?" then design-centered safety asks, "What is it about this system that made harm possible… or even likely?"

A design-informed perspective starts earlier. It asks how the system was arranged, what demands it placed on the people working within it, and where the fit between system design and actual work had begun to erode.

## From Active Errors to Latent Conditions

The work of James Reason and others fundamentally reshaped how safety professionals understood harm by directing attention away from isolated acts of failure and toward the conditions embedded within systems. Harm often reflects latent conditions that sit quietly within staffing structures, supervisory practices, physical layouts, technologies, communication pathways, and performance expectations long before an event occurs. These conditions may not produce immediate failure. They may instead be worked around, absorbed, or normalized over time [21].

That is part of their difficulty. A system condition can be risky without being dramatic. When teams compensate for it repeatedly, it becomes part of what ordinary work feels like. What should appear fragile may instead come to seem routine.

Reason's "Swiss Cheese Model" offered a metaphor for making this visible by showing how multiple layers of defense may weaken and align [21]. Its contribution was considerable, particularly in helping the field move away from simple blame narratives. Its limits, however, are increasingly apparent in contemporary healthcare. Clinical systems do not consist of fixed barriers and predictable gaps. They consist of moving relationships, competing demands, and changing contexts. Risk is shaped within those interactions.

In response, more dynamic frameworks have emerged. The Human Factors Analysis and Classification System (HFACS), originally developed in aviation and military domains, extends Reason's thinking by accounting for cognitive states, supervisory practices, organizational culture, and environmental constraints [22]. Rather than treating human error as a failure endpoint,

HFACS situates it within a broader sociotechnical system, recognizing that decisions made at leadership, policy, and design levels profoundly impact individual and team performance. When applied in healthcare, HFACS has enabled more nuanced analyses of patient safety events by highlighting how system-level conditions, such as productivity pressures, inadequate supervision, or poorly designed technologies, interact with human cognition and behavior to create highways to harm [23].

Together, these models reinforce a critical insight: harm is rarely the result of a single mistake or a single moment. It is more often the predictable outcome of systems that silently accumulate risk over time, until everyday work can no longer compensate for it. To address latent conditions, patient safety efforts must move past retrospective explanations toward approaches that surface hidden vulnerabilities before they converge, laying the groundwork for human-centered design strategies.

## Stakeholder Dissonance and Safety Blind Spots

Design problems often stem from mismatches between the assumptions of those designing the solution and the actual realities of end users. For example, in the adoption of health information technology, the views of nurses and other clinical staff are frequently underrepresented, resulting in workflow disruptions, effort duplication, and cognitive overload. When designers and users operate with different mental models of work, hidden drivers of unsafe care emerge [5].

Work-arounds are especially revealing in this context. Jane Fulton Suri used the term "thoughtless acts" to describe the improvised behaviors people adopt in response to poor design [24]. In healthcare, these may include storing supplies outside designated locations, hand-writing information that should be easy to retrieve electronically, or bypassing a formal step because it is too cumbersome to use under real conditions. Such behaviors are often categorized as noncompliance. They can also be read more usefully as evidence. They indicate where system design is asking users to choose between procedural purity and workable care.

## The Systemic Nature of Harm

Reframing harm as a design issue shifts the focus of patient safety away from isolated failures; these events are rarely the result of a single mistake or breakdown. They emerge from ongoing interactions among people, technologies, environments, and organizational structures, often in ways that remain invisible if patient safety investigations focus narrowly on individual actions or policy deviations.

Consider a delay in administering a time-sensitive medication. A traditional review may settle quickly on inattention, missed escalation, or failure to follow procedure. A design-centered lens, however, would reveal a more complex web of contributing factors: a medication dispensing interface that obscures critical information, packaging and labeling that increase the risk of selection errors, escalation pathways that are poorly defined or inconsistently applied, and staffing models that leave little margin for recovery under peak workload. Each factor alone may appear manageable, but together they create the conditions in which harm becomes not only possible, but increasingly likely. These interactions often fall outside the scope of conventional safety reviews, which are ill-equipped to capture how multiple system elements converge in real time.

Design-based analyses have proven particularly valuable in uncovering these latent, system-induced risks. In their examination of maternal safety, Sherman and colleagues applied design thinking across labor and delivery units in California to explore how environmental and procedural design influenced response during obstetric emergencies. Using on-site walkthroughs, stakeholder interviews, and simulation-based observations, the team identified inconsistencies in room layouts, delays in locating emergency equipment, and fragmented communication protocols. These design misalignments, though rarely flagged in standard safety audits, directly affected the speed and coordination of responses to maternal hemorrhage and neonatal distress [14].

Importantly, the study demonstrated that even technologically advanced, high-performing units were not immune to design-related risk. State-of-the-art facilities, when misaligned with the realities of clinical work, can inadvertently introduce friction, delay, and confusion at precisely the moments when clarity and coordination are most critical. By making these systemic interactions visible, a design-centered approach reframes harm not as an aberration, but as a predictable outcome of systems that have not been deliberately designed to support safe performance under stress.

### A Systems-Aware, Human-Centered Lens

Understanding harm as a consequence of system design opens a different set of responses. The question is no longer confined to whether individuals complied with policy or followed protocol. It extends to how systems make safe performance easier or harder under the conditions in which care is actually delivered.

Human-centered design approaches are valuable here because they require close engagement with the people using the system. Their aim is not simply to gather opinions, but to understand constraint, burden, adaptation, and unmet need in real settings. This moves patient safety work away from a model driven primarily by incident response and toward one oriented to iterative learning, early detection of fragility, and redesign grounded in practice.

## Design Thinking as a Safety Methodology

Design thinking is a structured approach to problem solving that begins with people's lived experience and works outward toward solutions. Originally developed in the fields of engineering and product design, it has since evolved into a multidisciplinary methodology used in business, education, social innovation, and increasingly, healthcare. Its appeal lies in its ability to navigate ambiguity, engage diverse stakeholders, and surface hidden knowledge, qualities often lacking in traditional healthcare improvement methods.

At its core, design thinking is grounded in five stages: empathize, define, ideate, prototype, and test (the d.school) [25]. These stages are not linear, but cyclical and overlapping, supporting cycles of learning.

*Empathize:* develop a deep understanding of user experience through interviews, shadowing, and immersion.
*Define:* synthesize findings to articulate key problems and unmet needs.
*Ideate:* generate a broad range of creative solutions through brainstorming and divergent thinking.
*Prototype:* build low-fidelity models to explore feasibility, usability, and user response.

## Test: Gather User Feedback to Refine and Evolve Solutions

The significance of the method lies less in the vocabulary of the model than in the stance it requires. Design thinking asks teams to observe before optimizing, to clarify the problem before institutionalizing a response, and to test interventions before scaling them.

## Complementing Traditional Improvement Approaches

In healthcare, design thinking is most useful when paired with existing quality improvement (QI) methodologies, including Lean, Six Sigma, and Plan-Do-Study-Act (PDSA) cycles, by addressing persistent limitations related to empathy, innovation, and context sensitivity.

Traditional QI approaches are highly effective when problems are well defined and processes are stable. Lean excels at identifying waste and inefficiency, Six Sigma focuses on reducing variation and defects, and PDSA supports iterative testing of incremental change. Together, these methods have driven important gains in reliability and standardization across healthcare systems.

However, many patient safety problems are not initially clear. They may present as delays, errors, or nonadherence, while the real issue lies in a mismatch between workflow, information flow, environment, and human capacity. The premature application of traditional optimization tools can result in well-executed solutions to the wrong problem. Design thinking targets this gap by emphasizing problem reframing, sensemaking, and exploration before solution development, creating space to interrogate assumptions that traditional QI methods commonly take for granted [26].

Design thinking helps uncover issues that are difficult to quantify or capture through existing metrics. By engaging directly with patients, families, and staff through interviews, observation, journey mapping, and co-creation, design methods surface emotional, cultural, and behavioral drivers that shape real-world performance. These insights often remain invisible in incident reports, dashboards, or time-motion studies, yet they exert a powerful influence over outcomes. Rather than replacing data-driven improvement, design thinking enriches it by expanding what counts as relevant evidence.

Crowe and colleagues observe that many improvement initiatives stall not because teams fail to execute change effectively but because they fail to identify the right problem to solve [11]. Design methods are particularly strong at this early, formative stage of improvement work. By grounding inquiry in lived experience and examining how work is actually performed rather than how it is imagined or prescribed, design thinking helps reveal foundational issues that traditional analytical approaches may overlook. Once these underlying needs and constraints are clarified, QI methodologies and tools can be applied more effectively to test, refine, and scale solutions that are both operationally sound and contextually appropriate.

Viewed together, design thinking and traditional QI form a complementary toolkit. Design thinking expands the problem space, surfaces hidden drivers of risk and resilience, and supports creative exploration. QI methods then provide the discipline, measurement, and rigor needed to implement and sustain change. When integrated thoughtfully, these approaches enable healthcare organizations to move beyond incremental optimization toward more meaningful, human-centered improvements in patient safety.

## Frameworks and Process Models

Beyond the d.school model, several established frameworks make design thinking usable in healthcare. Although they differ in form, they share a common function: they help teams examine difficult problems without moving too quickly to a preferred solution.

The *Double Diamond model* provides a clear visual representation of divergent and convergent thinking across four phases: discover, define, develop, and deliver [27]. In healthcare, this model is especially useful for resisting the impulse to jump to solutions. By explicitly separating exploration from decision-making, the Double Diamond creates space to broaden understanding of patient and clinician experiences before narrowing focus. This discipline helps teams avoid optimizing isolated processes while overlooking deeper systemic or experiential drivers of harm.

The *AHEAD framework* (approach to human-centered, evidence-driven adaptive design) responds to the unique demands of complex healthcare settings by integrating human-centered design with rigorous empirical methods [28]. AHEAD emphasizes the importance of grounding design work in high-quality evidence, including qualitative research, clinical data, and implementation science. This integration allows teams to move beyond anecdotal insight without losing sight of lived experience, ensuring that innovations are both contextually grounded and scientifically defensible. The framework is particularly well-suited for environments where safety, equity, and scalability are paramount.

*Codesign and participatory design approaches* extend design thinking further by redefining who participates in the creation of solutions. Rather than treating patients, families, and clinicians/staff as sources of data or end-stage reviewers, these approaches position them as equal partners throughout the design process [29]. By involving those who experience care firsthand in generating, testing, and refining interventions, codesign helps surface tacit knowledge, challenge unexamined assumptions, and build trust and ownership. In patient safety work, this shared authorship is especially critical, given that it aligns solutions with real-world constraints and reduces the likelihood of unintended consequences.

Collectively, these frameworks encourage structured creativity, rapid iteration, and context-specific learning, capabilities that are essential for addressing the complexity and variability of health systems. More importantly, they provide practical mechanisms for translating insight into action, enabling healthcare organizations to design safety interventions that are not only theoretically sound but also usable, adaptable, and resilient in practice.

## Mindsets and Cultural Shifts

Design thinking is not merely a collection of tools or techniques; it represents a fundamental shift in how problems are understood and how change is pursued. At its core, it is a mindset that values curiosity over certainty, humility over expertise, collaboration over hierarchy, and experimentation over premature optimization. Rather than assuming that complex challenges can be solved through analysis and mapping alone, design thinking invites sustained inquiry into how systems are actually experienced by the people who inhabit them.

In practice, this mindset disrupts traditional hierarchical norms by broadening who is invited into problem framing and decision-making. Patients, families, frontline clinicians, and support staff are no longer positioned solely as data sources or recipients of change, but as partners in sensemaking and solution development. Design thinking places particular emphasis on making experience visible through visual and experiential methods, such as journey mapping, storyboarding, role-play, and simulation. These tools help teams move beyond abstract descriptions of work to a shared, tangible understanding of how care unfolds across time, space, and roles. By drawing on insights from anthropology, psychology, human factors, and systems engineering, design thinking integrates multiple ways of knowing to illuminate dimensions of safety that are often overlooked by traditional approaches.

Adopting this way of working is rarely comfortable, however. Design thinking requires organizations to tolerate ambiguity, surface inconvenient truths, and question long-standing assumptions about efficiency, control, and expertise. In healthcare settings, where accountability structures are tightly coupled to performance metrics and regulatory compliance, creating space for exploration can feel risky. Meaningful implementation often depends on explicit leadership and institutional support, cultural adaptation, and the space to engage in iterative learning, even when early efforts do not yield immediate or easily quantifiable results.

When these conditions are present, however, design-based approaches can fundamentally alter how organizations learn and improve. Studies across sectors suggest that human-centered design is associated with higher levels of engagement, stronger cross-disciplinary collaboration, and solutions that are more closely aligned with user needs and real-world constraints [12]. In healthcare, this translates into interventions that clinicians are more likely to adopt, patients are more likely to trust, and systems are more likely to sustain over time. Ultimately, design thinking offers not just a method for innovation, but a way of cultivating adaptive capacity, enabling healthcare organizations to evolve in response to complexity rather than react to failure.

## Evidence Across Sectors and Settings

The application of design thinking to healthcare is no longer speculative. A growing body of empirical research, implementation studies, and cross-sector adaptation demonstrates the value of human-centered design for solving complex patient safety problems. From intensive care to ambulatory screening, from professional education to digital systems, these interventions reflect a shared insight: systems improve when they are reimagined through the lived experiences of users.

## High-Pressure Clinical Environments

In high-acuity environments such as intensive care units (ICUs), design thinking has been used to enhance workflow, communication, and patient experience. Krolikowski et al. describe how a multidisciplinary team in a U.S. academic medical center ICU applied design thinking to address clinician burnout, information bottlenecks, and fragmented care coordination. Using ethnographic shadowing and collaborative workshops, the team cocreated low-fidelity prototypes of redesigned workstations, visual care plans, and communication boards. These were tested in situ with nurses, residents, and attendings, revealing that even minor changes, such as shared rounding tools and reorganized team spaces, could reduce documentation redundancy, minimize interruptions, and improve staff morale. The project demonstrated that iterative prototyping with frontline teams could yield high-impact, sustainable improvements in complex critical care settings [13].

Similarly, Sherman et al. applied a design lens to examine heterogeneity across labor and delivery units in California, finding that differences in physical space design, access to emergency equipment, and handoff communication protocols significantly influenced maternal and neonatal outcomes. Their work emphasized the need for adaptable safety infrastructure that reflects clinical variability, not rigid adherence to standardized checklists [14].

## Education and Workforce Development

Design thinking also supports healthcare professional development, especially in building competencies that are difficult to teach through didactic methods: empathy, teamwork, systems thinking, and adaptability. Moon and Chang conducted a quasi-experimental study involving undergraduate nursing students across multiple institutions in South Korea. The intervention group received patient safety education rooted in design thinking: engaging in empathy interviews, scenario mapping, and solution sketching focused on real clinical challenges. Compared to peers trained via conventional case-based learning, students in the design thinking cohort showed significantly greater gains in safety knowledge, communication confidence, and professional identity formation. Notably, participants also expressed a stronger appreciation for interprofessional collaboration and systems-level awareness, key traits often underdeveloped in early clinical education [30].

At the system level, Hinic and Kowalski used design thinking to expand an evidence-based practice (EBP) education program for over 4000 nurses across seven hospitals. Their dual-track approach- offering both a yearlong EBP Scholars fellowship and flexible webinar-based learning- was informed directly by user feedback about scheduling needs, mentorship gaps, and digital access [31].

### Digital Health and Equity

Design thinking has proven especially valuable in addressing digital access and health equity. Levander et al. used human-centered design to co-develop a telehealth interface tailored to the needs of low-income, predominantly non-English-speaking patients in urban US clinics. Through design sprints and contextual inquiry, they uncovered that shared phone access, limited broadband, and visual literacy constituted significant barriers to traditional digital health platforms. The team cocreated solutions such as simplified user flows, culturally tailored visuals, and low-data usage video tools, all piloted with community health workers and patient advocates. The result was a telehealth prototype that increased completion rates for scheduled virtual visits and improved user satisfaction, highlighting the role of HCD in advancing health equity [10].

In Brazil, a machine learning-enabled trigger system for detecting ambulatory care harm was developed through design thinking methods. Rather than relying solely on retrospective claims data or top-down algorithms, they engaged clinicians in codesign workshops to define meaningful “trigger” signals: patterns suggesting possible harm events like missed follow-ups or diagnostic delays. This participatory approach led to higher clinician trust in the AI outputs and improved integration of the alerts into clinical workflows, reinforcing that predictive analytics can be enhanced through collaborative, context-sensitive design [32].

## Cross-Industry Lessons: Oil, Insurance, and Aviation

The principles of human-centered design are not exclusive to healthcare; they have proven effective in a variety of complex service environments where risk, emotion, and system fragmentation cause significant challenges. Design thinking's origins in industrial design have enabled valuable cross-sector learning. In the oil and gas industry, HFACS-based frameworks adapted from aviation revealed how communication breakdowns, poor supervision, and organizational climate contribute to catastrophic events, insights transferable to healthcare's high-stakes environments [33].

In the insurance industry, Gauthier and Therrien's work revealed that employee disengagement and internal inefficiencies often mirrored the client-facing issues the company sought to solve. Using service design tools like journey mapping and persona creation, they worked with claims adjusters and service reps to redesign workflows, digital interfaces, and support tools. The result was not only improved customer satisfaction scores but also a measurable reduction in processing time and burnout rates—offering a valuable parallel for healthcare, where internal user experience can be as critical as patient-facing systems [34].

These cross-sector experiences highlight a central insight: safety and quality emerge not solely from compliance or control, but from systems designed to align with the real needs and constraints of the people who use them. Whether in oil refineries or insurance call centers, performance failures often reflect design mismatches rather than individual shortcomings. For healthcare, this highlights the imperative to treat internal workflow design, staff experience, and organizational culture not as secondary concerns, but as critical dimensions of patient safety strategy.

## What the Shift Requires from Leaders and Systems

The successful integration of design thinking into healthcare safety is not merely a technical exercise; it is an organizational and cultural transformation. Design thinking invites institutions to reframe their relationship to risk, failure, and innovation. It challenges entrenched hierarchies, promotes cross-disciplinary collaboration, and repositions patients and frontline workers as cocreators of safety, not passive recipients of interventions. For design thinking to take root, leadership must actively cultivate conditions in which psychological safety, experimentation, and learning are not just permitted but institutionalized.

### Psychological Safety and Innovation

Psychological safety—the shared belief that team members can take interpersonal risks without fear of humiliation or retribution—is foundational to high-performing healthcare teams and a critical precondition for innovation. A 2023 integrative review by Edmondson and Bransby identifies psychological safety as essential to adaptive performance, particularly in dynamic settings like healthcare, where collaboration, communication, and learning are continual and interdependent [35]. In environments where staff feel unsafe to speak up or question processes, the kind of honest feedback and insight needed for human-centered design rarely emerges.

Leaders must tolerate ambiguity and divergent thinking while actively modeling curiosity and empathy. The design process inherently involves failure, reframing, and iteration. Organizational cultures accustomed to linear planning and fixed metrics may struggle to accommodate this mindset unless senior leaders explicitly endorse exploratory work and protect it from premature evaluation [36].

## Flattening Hierarchies and Enabling Co-creation

Traditional healthcare structures tend to reinforce steep hierarchies across disciplines, roles, and departments, often privileging formal authority and technical expertise over lived experience. While these hierarchies can support accountability and specialization, they can also fragment understanding and limit the flow of insight across the system. Design thinking challenges this fragmentation by emphasizing radical collaboration: intentionally bringing together patients, families, clinicians, administrators, designers, and support staff to jointly define problems and cocreate solutions. In doing so, it reframes improvement not as something imposed from above, but as a shared endeavor grounded in collective sensemaking.

This collaborative orientation reflects a deeper recognition that safety is not solely a technical outcome of protocols, checklists, or compliance mechanisms. Rather, safety emerges from the quality of relationships within the system, shaped by trust, communication, psychological safety, and the ability of individuals and teams to learn together. When diverse perspectives are invited into problem framing, hidden assumptions are surfaced, power dynamics are softened, and solutions are more likely to reflect the realities of everyday work. Design thinking creates structured spaces where hierarchy gives way to curiosity and where differences in role or status become sources of insight rather than barriers to participation.

The practical impact of this approach is illustrated by the work of Casarett and colleagues, who applied a hybrid implementation model combining RE-AIM (reach, effectiveness, adoption, implementation, maintenance) with design thinking to scale a goals-of-care documentation initiative across multiple departments. Rather than relying solely on top-down mandates or standardized templates, the team engaged clinicians and staff through rapid ethnography and participatory workshops to codesign electronic medical record (EMR) templates, clinician prompts, and training modules that respected time constraints while enhancing documentation quality. Journey mapping was used to visualize patient conversations and team experiences, revealing points of friction, emotional burden, and missed opportunities.

By making these interactions visible and open to collective redesign, the initiative identified unintended burdens early and adjusted interventions accordingly. The result was improved documentation fidelity, increased clinician confidence in advance care planning, and greater alignment between system expectations and clinical practice [37]. More broadly, the study demonstrates how design thinking can translate collaborative ideals into measurable outcomes, offering a compelling model for how inclusive, human-centered approaches can strengthen both the technical and relational foundations of patient safety.

## Designing for the System, Not the Hero

One of the most enduring and culturally reinforced myths in healthcare is the "hero narrative": the belief that patient safety depends primarily on the vigilance, dedication, and resilience of exceptional individuals. Clinicians are celebrated for catching errors, working around broken processes, and absorbing system strain through personal sacrifice. While individual resilience and professionalism are unquestionably important, reliance on heroism is inherently fragile. It assumes that people can indefinitely compensate for poorly designed systems, escalating complexity, and chronic resource constraints, an expectation that is neither humane nor sustainable.

When safety depends on individual vigilance alone, it becomes vulnerable to fatigue, cognitive overload, and burnout. Over time, the very adaptations that allow clinicians to keep patients safe in the moment can obscure deeper system flaws, normalizing workarounds and masking risk rather than eliminating it. In this sense, adverse events could be framed as personal failures, even when they arise from predictable system conditions that exceed human limits. Design thinking challenges this logic by shifting the locus of responsibility from individuals to the systems in which they work. Rather than asking people to be endlessly resilient, it asks how systems can be deliberately designed to support safe performance under real-world conditions.

Design-led approaches reorient safety efforts toward creating environments, tools, and workflows that make the right action the easy action. In clinical settings ranging from neonatal resuscitation rooms to intensive care unit (ICU) charting stations, design interventions have moved attention away from individual memory and improvisation toward environmental cues, shared mental models, and team-based coordination. Examples include standardized room layouts that reduce search time during emergencies, visual displays that support shared situational awareness, and documentation interfaces that align with clinical reasoning rather than interrupt it.

These design shifts do not diminish the role of human expertise; rather, they amplify it by reducing unnecessary cognitive burden and supporting timely, coordinated action. By embedding safety into the physical and digital environment, design-led improvements replace reliance on heroics with systems that anticipate human limitations and leverage human strengths. In doing so, they make safe action more intuitive, visible, and reliable, enabling clinicians to focus their attention on clinical judgment and patient care rather than system navigation [13].

## Strategic Alignment and Institutional Embedding

For design thinking to move beyond episodic projects and isolated innovation efforts, it must be deliberately embedded within an organization's core strategy for quality, safety, and operational performance. When design is treated as an ad hoc capability, its impact remains local and fragile. When it is institutionalized, it becomes a force multiplier, improving the effectiveness of existing investments in clinical operations, digital transformation, and capital planning. Strategic alignment requires more than endorsement; it requires governance structures that give design authority, accountability, and continuity. This includes establishing formal roles, such as a chief design officer or embedded design leadership within quality and safety functions, funding dedicated design capacity, and integrating design-informed indicators into enterprise dashboards alongside traditional performance metrics.

Critically, organizations must reconcile the timelines of design work with existing performance and growth cycles. Design thinking is most valuable upstream, before capital is deployed, technologies are purchased, or policies are locked in. At this stage, insight-gathering and prototyping may not immediately translate into measurable ROI, yet they materially reduce downstream risk. By identifying misalignment early, whether between workflows and technology, staff capability and policy expectations, or physical space and care delivery models, design thinking prevents the far more expensive consequences of rework, underutilized assets, clinician disengagement, and failed adoption. From a growth and margin perspective, this is not a delay in value creation; it is a form of risk mitigation and capital protection.

Health systems that have scaled design capacity demonstrate that it strengthens, rather than competes with, operational discipline. Organizations such as the Veterans Health Administration and Kaiser Permanente have made design a durable part of their operating model, informing policy, facility planning, and technology decisions. At Kaiser, the Garfield Innovation Center enables live prototyping of care environments, allowing layouts, digital displays, and workflows to be tested with frontline staff prior to system-wide rollout, reducing adoption risk and downstream cost [38].

From a growth perspective, institutionalized design capacity improves execution certainty. It increases the likelihood that large-scale initiatives will be adopted, sustained, and scaled, protecting both operating margin and strategic momentum. It also accelerates learning across the enterprise, enabling organizations to adapt faster in the face of market, workforce, and regulatory volatility. In this sense, design thinking is not an innovation luxury; it is a strategic capability that strengthens the return on existing investments, reduces avoidable failure, and supports durable growth in complex health systems.

## Conclusion

Patient safety now faces a more difficult task than the field first imagined. Preventable harm is no longer adequately understood as the result of isolated breakdowns requiring better detection and correction. It is also shaped by how care systems are configured, how clinicians and patients move through them, and how much hidden adaptation is required to keep those systems functioning.

Safety, then, is a matter of design as well as analysis. Retrospective investigation remains essential, but it cannot bear the full burden of learning in environments where fragility accumulates gradually and often quietly. The more demanding task is to recognize the conditions under which failure becomes more likely while there is still time to alter them.

That requires methods able to examine experience, make weak points in ordinary work more visible, and test safer arrangements before they harden into policy or routine. It also requires a broader understanding of what counts as safety knowledge. Event reports and causal analysis remain important, but they do not fully reveal how systems sustain safety, absorb strain, or edge closer to breakdown while outwardly continuing to function.

## References


1. Kohn LT, Corrigan JM, Donaldson MS, editors. To err is human: building a safer health system. Washington (DC): National Academy Press; 2000. https://doi.org/10.17226/9728.
2. James JT. A new, evidence-based estimate of patient harms associated with hospital care. J Patient Saf. 2013;9(3):122–8. https://doi.org/10.1097/PTS.0b013e3182948a69.
3. Makary MA, Daniel M. Medical error—the third leading cause of death in the US. BMJ. 2016;353:i2139. https://doi.org/10.1136/bmj.i2139.
4. World Health Organization. Patient safety fact file. Geneva: WHO; 2023. Available from: https://www.who.int/news-room/fact-sheets/detail/patient-safety
5. Samaras EA, Real SD, Curtis AM, Meunier TS. Recognizing nurse stakeholder dissonance as a critical determinant of patient safety in new healthcare information technologies. Work. 2012;41:1904–10. https://doi.org/10.3233/WOR-2012-0406-1904.

6. Bhattacharyya O, Blumenthal D, Stoddard R, Mansell L, Mossman K, Schneider E. Redesigning care: adapting new improvement methods to achieve person-centered care. BMJ Qual Saf. 2019;28(3):242–8. https://doi.org/10.1136/bmjqs-2018-008208.
7. Ash JS, Sittig DF, Dykstra R, Campbell EM, Guappone KP, Dykstra RH. Some unintended consequences of clinical decision support systems. AMIA Annu Symp Proc. 2007;2007:26–30.
8. Wu AW, Lipshutz AK, Pronovost PJ. Effectiveness and efficiency of root cause analysis in medicine. JAMA. 2008;299(6):685–7. https://doi.org/10.1001/jama.299.6.685.
9. Hollnagel E. Safety-I and safety-II: the past and future of safety management. Farnham: Ashgate; 2014. https://doi.org/10.1201/9781315607511.
10. Levander XA, VanDerSchaaf H, Barragan VG, Choxi H, Hoffman A, Morgan E, et al. The role of human-centered design in healthcare innovation: a digital health equity case study. J Gen Intern Med. 2024;39(4):690–5. https://doi.org/10.1007/s11606-023-08500-0.
11. Crowe B, Gaulton JS, Minor N, Asch DA, Eyet J, Rainosek E, et al. To improve quality, leverage design. BMJ Qual Saf. 2022;31(2):70–4. https://doi.org/10.1136/bmjqs-2021-013605.
12. Roschetal N, Tiberius V, Kraus S. Design thinking for innovation: context factors, process, and outcomes. Eur J Innov Manag. 2023;26(7):160–76. https://doi.org/10.1108/EJIM-03-2022-0164.
13. Krolikowski KA, Mengxue B, Baggott CM, Khorzad R, Holl JL, Kruser JM. Design thinking to improve healthcare delivery in the intensive care unit: promises, pitfalls, and lessons learned. J Crit Care. 2022;69:153999. https://doi.org/10.1016/j.jcrc.2022.153999.
14. Sherman JP, Hedli LC, Kristensen-Cabrera AI, Lipman SS, Schwandt D, Lee HC, et al. Understanding the heterogeneity of labor and delivery units: using design thinking to assess environmental factors that contribute to safety in childbirth. Am J Perinatol. 2020;37(6):638–46. https://doi.org/10.1055/s-0039-168549.
15. Cook RI, Render M, Woods DD. Gaps in the continuity of care and progress on patient safety. BMJ. 2000;320(7237):791–4. https://doi.org/10.1136/bmj.320.7237.791.
16. Peerally MF, Carr S, Waring J, Dixon-Woods M. The problem with root cause analysis. BMJ Qual Saf. 2017;26(5):417–22. https://doi.org/10.1136/bmjqs-2016-005511.
17. Martin-Delgado J, Martinez-Garcia A, Aranaz JM, Valencia-Martin JL, Mira JJ. How much of root cause analysis translates into improved patient safety: a systematic review. Med Princ Pract. 2020;29(6):524–31. https://doi.org/10.1159/000508677.
18. Braithwaite J, Wears RL, Hollnagel E. Resilient health care: turning patient safety on its head. Int J Qual Health Care. 2015;27(5):418–20. https://doi.org/10.1093/intqhc/mzv063.

19. Dixon-Woods M, McNicol S, Martin G. Ten challenges in improving quality in healthcare: lessons from the Health Foundation's program evaluations and relevant literature. BMJ Qual Saf. 2012;21(10):876–84. https://doi.org/10.1136/bmjqs-2011-000760.
20. Coles E, Anderson J, Maxwell M, Harris F, Gray N, Milner G, MacGillivray S. The influence of contextual factors on healthcare quality improvement initiatives: a realist review. Syst Rev. 2020;9(1):94. https://doi.org/10.1186/s13643-020-01344-3.
21. Reason J. Human error: models and management. BMJ. 2000;320(7237):768–70. https://doi.org/10.1136/bmj.320.7237.768.
22. Lee J, Huang C, Sie Y, Yang P, Su C, Chang J. Applying the human factors analysis and classification system within root cause analysis to prevent medical errors and enhancing patient safety culture: insights from a medical center. Int J Qual Health Care. 2025;37(1):mzaf009. https://doi.org/10.1093/intqhc/mzaf009.
23. Jalali M, Dehghan H, Habibi E, Khakzad N. Application of human factor analysis and classification system (HFACS) model to the prevention of medical errors and adverse events: a systematic review. Int J Prev Med. 2023;14:1–11. https://doi.org/10.4103/ijpvm.ijpvm_123_22.
24. Suri JF, IDEO. Thoughtless acts?: observations on intuitive design. San Francisco: Chronicle Books; 2005.
25. Brown T. Change by design: how design thinking transforms organizations and inspires innovation. Boston: Harvard Business Press; 2009.
26. Barr E, Brannan GD. Quality improvement methods (LEAN, PDSA, SIX SIGMA). In: StatPearls [Internet]. Treasure Island: StatPearls Publishing; 2024. [cited 2026]. Available from: https://www.ncbi.nlm.nih.gov/books/NBK599556/.
27. Design Council. The double diamond: a universally accepted depiction of the design process. London: Design Council; 2019. Available from: https://www.designcouncil.org.uk/our-work/skills-learning/tools-frameworks/design-process/
28. Fischer M, Safaeinili N, Haverfield M, Brown-Johnson C, Zionts D, Zulman D. Approach to human-centered, evidence-driven adaptive design (AHEAD) for health care interventions: a proposed framework. J Gen Intern Med. 2021;36(4):1041–8. https://doi.org/10.1007/s11606-020-06451-4.
29. Bate P, Robert G. Experience-based design: from redesigning the system around the patient to co-designing services with the patient. Qual Saf Health Care. 2006;15(5):307–10. https://doi.org/10.1136/qshc.2005.016527.
30. Moon S, Chang SJ. Comparing the effects of patient safety education using design thinking and case-based learning on nursing students' competence and professional socialization: a quasi-experimental design. Heliyon. 2024;10(9):e29942. https://doi.org/10.1016/j.heliyon.2024.e29942.

31. Hinic K, Kowalski MO. Use of design thinking to grow the reach and relevance of evidence-based practice education across a health care system. J Contin Educ Nurs. 2023;54(8):360–6. https://doi.org/10.3928/00220124-20230711-06.
32. Herrera CN, Gimenes FR, Herrera JP, Cavalli R. Development of automated triggers in ambulatory settings in Brazil: protocol for a machine learning-based design thinking study. JMIR Res Protoc. 2024;13:e55466. https://doi.org/10.2196/55466.
33. Nwankwo CD, Arewa AO, Theophilus SC, Esenowo VN. Analysis of accidents caused by human factors in the oil and gas industry using the HFACS-OGI framework. Int J Occup Saf Ergon. 2022;28(3):1642–54. https://doi.org/10.1080/10803548.2021.1916238.
34. Iriarte I, Alberdi A, Urrutia E, Justel D. Beyond customer satisfaction: supporting organisational change through service design. A case study in the insurance industry. Des J. 2017;20:424–34. https://doi.org/10.1080/14606925.2017.1352950.
35. Edmondson AC, Bransby DP. Psychological safety comes of age: observed themes in an established literature. Annu Rev Organ Psychol Organ Behav. 2023;10:55–78. https://doi.org/10.1146/annurev-orgpsych-120920-055217.
36. Norman D. The design of everyday things. New York (NY): Basic Books; 2013.
37. Casarett D, Lakis K, Ma JE, Fischer J, Ibrahim S. Using design thinking to promote goals of care conversations with seriously ill patients. J Pain Symptom Manag. 2023;66(2):275–81. https://doi.org/10.1016/j.jpainsymman.2023.04.010.
38. Bhattacharyya O, Mossman K, Gustafsson L, Schneider EC. Innovating health care: learning what works, where, and why. JAMA. 2018;320(15):1451–2. https://doi.org/10.1001/jama.2018.14020.

# Design Thinking Unpacked

# 2

## Introduction

Design thinking is frequently invoked in healthcare, but much less often defined with precision. In some settings, the term is reduced to brainstorming, workshop facilitation, or a set of innovation rituals detached from serious clinical work. That reduction is one reason the method is often met with skepticism. In safety-critical environments, any approach that appears vague, aesthetic, or loosely applied will struggle to earn trust.

The issue is not whether design thinking sounds appealing. The issue is whether it offers a disciplined way of working with problems that are difficult to define in advance, shaped by multiple interacting conditions, and experienced differently across the people who move through them. Many patient safety challenges take exactly this form. They are not always reducible to one broken step in a process. They may involve competing priorities, poorly aligned technologies, unclear ownership, fragmented information, or burdens that are distributed unevenly across clinicians, patients, and families.

Under those conditions, improvement can falter even when the intention is sound and the execution is earnest. Teams may move quickly to intervention without having fully clarified the nature of the problem they are trying to solve. They may optimize one part of the system while leaving the larger source of difficulty largely


K. Rasmussen, *Rethinking Patient Safety*,
https://doi.org/10.1007/978-3-032-26054-3_2

intact. They may also rely too heavily on methods that assume stability and definitional clarity when neither is actually present.

Design thinking is relevant here because it introduces discipline at an earlier stage of inquiry. It slows the move from problem recognition to solution selection just enough to allow closer observation, broader participation, and more careful framing. That does not make it less rigorous than traditional improvement methods. In some cases, it makes rigor possible where premature certainty would otherwise narrow the work too soon.

## Core Principles of Design Thinking

Design thinking is often described as a process, but its coherence depends on a set of underlying principles. These principles shape how problems are approached, what kinds of evidence are taken seriously, and how teams move from observation to intervention. Although design thinking emerged from product and industrial design, its core commitments have been adapted across healthcare contexts, where uncertainty, vulnerability, and system complexity are central features of the work. Across the relevant literature, several principles appear consistently: empathy, iteration, co-creation, tolerance for ambiguity, and systems awareness [1, 2].

Empathy is the foundational principle of design thinking. It redirects inquiry toward the lived experience of the people within a system. In healthcare, this includes patients, family caregivers, clinicians, and staff. The point is not simply to cultivate sensitivity but to understand how care is actually encountered and where burdens, gaps, and frustrations accumulate. Recent work in nursing and health services research has shown that empathy-based methods can reveal emotional demands, inequities, and forms of process friction that are often overlooked when analysis begins and ends with performance metrics [3, 4]. Empathic fieldwork methods such as shadowing, narrative elicitation, and experience mapping are now common tools in health innovation settings [2].

Iteration is equally important. Design thinking does not assume that the first formulation of a solution will be sufficient. It depends instead on repeated cycles of making, testing, and refining. In healthcare education and practice, this orientation has been associated with greater adaptability, stronger confidence in problem solving, and increased willingness to revise an intervention in response to what is learned through use [4, 5]. This differs from more linear models in which failure is treated as evidence that a plan was flawed from the outset. Within design thinking, small failure is part of disciplined learning.

Co-creation is another defining principle. Design thinking differs from more traditional models of improvement in that it treats users as participants in design rather than as recipients of change. This is especially important in patient safety work, where interventions developed without the sustained involvement of frontline clinicians, patients, or caregivers often fail when they encounter real conditions. Reviews of codesign in healthcare have linked meaningful participation to greater uptake, stronger relevance, and more robust implementation [3, 6].

Tolerance for ambiguity is also central. Rather than rushing to solve predefined problems, it encourages reframing, asking, "Are we solving the right problem?" This principle is consistent with cognitive psychology research on premature closure and bias in clinical decision-making. It is also supported by case examples where the design process shifted project goals from surface solutions (e.g., enforcing protocols) to upstream system redesign (e.g., rethinking layout or communication tools) [2, 7].

Systems awareness completes the set. Design thinking assumes that behavior is shaped by a web of interacting conditions that include technologies, environments, rules, relationships, and cultural expectations. This makes it compatible with human factors engineering and sociotechnical systems theory, though it places greater emphasis on lived experience and usability. Recent design-oriented studies in health settings have shown how changes in environment, workflow visibility, and information design can influence safety-related behavior without relying solely on additional training or enforcement [5, 8].

Together, these principles form the ethical and methodological spine of design thinking in healthcare. Their value lies not in their novelty but in the discipline they introduce into how complex problems are seen, studied, and addressed.

## Translating Design Thinking Into Healthcare Safety

Principles become useful in practice when they are supported by models that organize inquiry and action. In patient safety work, where problems are rarely linear and solutions must function under real-world constraints, such models provide a structured way to move from observation to intervention.

### The Double Diamond Model

One of the most widely referenced models in design thinking is the Double Diamond, developed by the UK Design Council [9, 10]. The model provides a clear visual representation of alternating phases of divergent and convergent thinking, offering a shared language for exploring problems broadly before narrowing focus and committing to action. While the Double Diamond originated outside of healthcare, its underlying logic has been influential across industries characterized by complexity and uncertainty.

The value of the model in patient safety lies in the distinction it forces between understanding the problem and acting on it. In healthcare, those two forms of work are often compressed into one. Once a safety concern becomes visible, there is understandable pressure to act quickly. Corrective action may be necessary, especially when immediate stabilization is required. The difficulty arises when the need to respond becomes indistinguishable from the need to understand. The Double Diamond preserves that distinction.

At a conceptual level, the model helps teams resist premature closure. It also provides a useful language for differentiating exploration from decision-making. This is particularly important in patient safety work, where the urgency of an event can encourage fast convergence on interventions that are visible, documentable, and institutionally familiar, but not necessarily effective (Fig. 2.1).

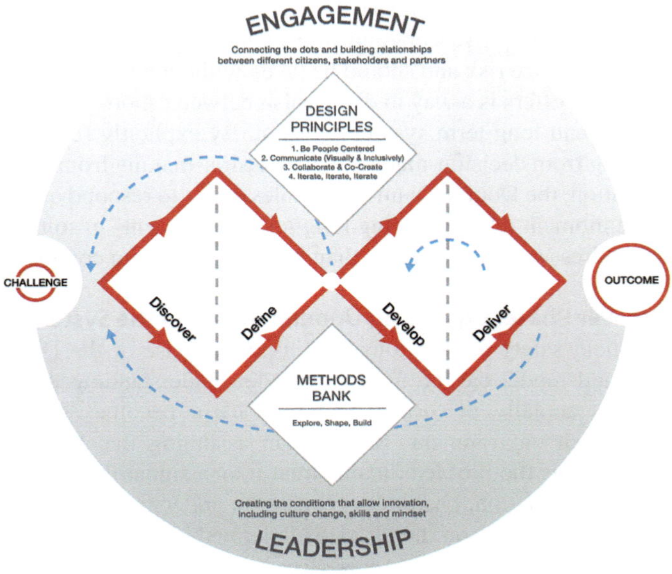


**Fig. 2.1** The double diamond model of design thinking developed by the UK Design Council, illustrating cycles of divergent and convergent thinking across four phases. Reproduced under the Creative Commons Attribution 4.0 International (CC BY 4.0) license. https://creativecommons.org/licenses/by/4.0/

## Applying the Double Diamond in Patient Safety Work

The Double Diamond is especially valuable in patient safety because it guards against a common failure mode: premature solution lock-in. Following a safety event, healthcare teams are understandably motivated to ensure that the error never occurs again. In this urgency, organizations often move directly from incident to intervention, implementing feasible but frequently low-impact responses such as additional training, new checklists, or policy reminders. While these actions may demonstrate responsiveness, they are often selected before the system dynamics that produced the harm are fully understood.

The Double Diamond does not advocate for delay or inaction. Immediate corrective steps and stopgap measures are often necessary to stabilize risk and should be taken without hesitation. What the model offers is a way to distinguish between short-term stabilization and long-term system redesign. By explicitly separating learning from decision-making, and decision-making from implementation, the Double Diamond enables teams to respond quickly in the moment while avoiding long-term investments in solutions that address symptoms rather than underlying system conditions.

#### Discover Phase: Expanding Understanding of the System

In patient safety applications, the discover phase of the Double Diamond model can be used to broaden understanding of how work is actually performed and how harm becomes possible within that environment. Rather than assuming that the event itself reveals the problem, teams treat it as a signal that calls for closer examination. Discovery focuses on understanding work as done *in the real world*, not work as imagined [10].

Typical activities during this phase include direct observation across shifts and roles, brief interviews with frontline clinicians and, when relevant, patients or caregivers, and review of artifacts such as order sets, documentation flows, physical room layouts, and communication tools. The goal is not to identify a single cause but to surface patterns, tensions, and constraints that shape behavior under real-world conditions. Outputs from this phase often include workflow maps, identification of recurring workarounds, and early hypotheses related to cognitive demand, information visibility, staffing, or environmental design.

#### Define Phase: Reframing the Safety Problem

The define phase of the Double Diamond model marks the first convergence [10]. Here, teams synthesize observations into a problem statement that can support design work. This step often changes the focus of the entire effort. Problems initially described in terms of noncompliance or individual error are frequently reframed as mismatches among tools, workflows, expectations, and human capacity.

Effective problem statements focus on *system needs* rather than individual behavior, specifying who is affected, under what conditions, and why existing structures fail to support safe performance. This reframing helps ensure that subsequent interventions target leverage points within the system rather than reinforcing compliance-based solutions that are unlikely to hold under pressure.

### Develop Phase: Exploring and Testing System Responses

The develop phase reopens the space of possibility. Teams generate multiple possible responses to the defined problem and begin testing them through rough, low-risk forms. This phase emphasizes learning through making rather than selecting a single "best" solution prematurely [10]. In patient safety contexts, prototypes might include workflow changes, environmental cues, information displays, role clarification tools, or low-fidelity technology mock-ups (wireframes, drawings, etc.).

This phase of experimentation focuses on usability, feasibility, and unintended consequences rather than outcomes alone. Prototypes are assessed under realistic conditions to understand how they interact with existing work patterns and constraints in a controlled approach. This allows teams to identify risk early, when change is still reversible, and to refine interventions before they are embedded in policy, technology, or physical space.

### Deliver Phase: Implementing with Feedback and Learning

The final convergence occurs in the deliver phase, where a refined intervention is piloted and, if successful, prepared for scale [10]. In patient safety work, this phase is most effective when it includes clear adoption measures, balancing metrics, and structured feedback loops. Rather than treating implementation as an endpoint, the Double Diamond model frames it as the beginning of a learning cycle, allowing interventions to evolve as they encounter the full complexity of everyday use.

## Adapting the Double Diamond for Patient Safety

In healthcare, the Double Diamond often needs adaptation because patient safety work unfolds under conditions that do not allow neat separation between correction and redesign. Clinical environments demand immediate stabilization alongside longer-term redesign, and safety interventions must function under conditions of time pressure, cognitive load, and variability. For this reason, the model should be adapted to explicitly distinguish between actions taken to reduce immediate risk and design work aimed at reshaping the system over time.

An adapted model retains the core logic of double divergence and convergence while incorporating patient safety-specific considerations, including the role of stopgap measures, the influence of human workload, and the need for ongoing adaptation after implementation. By making these elements explicit, the framework provides a practical guide for safety leaders and improvement teams seeking to apply design thinking rigorously without sacrificing responsiveness.

### A Case Example

To illustrate how the Double Diamond model can be adapted and applied in practice, consider a common and high-risk scenario: the delayed administration of time-critical medications in a hospital setting. Such delays are frequently identified through safety event reporting and quality key performance indicators (KPIs) and are often addressed through reminders, education, or policy reinforcement. While these actions may reduce visible noncompliance, they rarely resolve the underlying conditions that make delays likely under routine operating pressures.

### Discover: Understanding System Conditions

In the discover phase, the delay itself is treated as a signal rather than the problem to be solved. Inquiry begins by examining how medication administration unfolds in *real* clinical conditions, particularly during periods of high workload or interruption. Observations and interviews with nurses across shifts reveal recurring patterns: competing clinical priorities, frequent interruptions during medication preparation, fragmented information, and uncertainty about escalation expectations when medications are delayed for clinically defensible reasons.

Shadowing experiences and workflow mapping highlight additional constraints that are not captured in policy. For example, nurses describe needing to navigate multiple screens to confirm medication timing, reconcile conflicting alerts, and document administration, all while responding to call lights and coordinating with providers. Informal workarounds, such as batching documentation or relying on memory rather than real-time prompts, emerge as adaptive strategies…not as rule violations. These insights surface latent system conditions: cognitive overload, interface design issues, and misalignment between task demands and staffing patterns.

### Define: Reframing the Safety Problem

During the define phase, insights from the discovery phase are synthesized into a reframed problem statement. Rather than defining the issue as failure to administer medications on time, the safety challenge is articulated as a system that does not reliably support timely action under variable conditions. The problem is reframed to focus on information visibility, prioritization under interruption, and unclear escalation pathways…not individual performance.

A refined problem statement might read: *Clinicians need a way to identify, prioritize, and escalate time-critical medications during high-interruption periods without increasing cognitive burden or documentation workload.* This reframing shifts the focus from compliance to support and establishes clear design constraints, including the need to function during peak workload periods, avoid additional clicks, and accommodate clinically appropriate delays.

### Develop: Designing and Testing Interventions

In the develop phase, teams explore multiple intervention concepts rather than landing prematurely on a single solution. Options may include redesigned medication administration record (MAR) views that visually surface time-critical medications, environmental cues that signal priority tasks during medication preparation, simplified escalation prompts embedded in existing workflows, or role clarification tools that support team-based coverage during peak demand.

Low-fidelity prototypes are created and tested. Paper mockups of revised electronic views, simulated handoffs during medication administration, and brief role-play scenarios allow clinicians to interact with proposed changes under realistic conditions. Testing focuses not only on whether delays decrease but also on whether interventions reduce cognitive load, integrate smoothly into workflows, and avoid causing new risks or workarounds. Some concepts may be discarded after early testing reveals they add additional burden, while others are refined based on frontline feedback.

#### Deliver: Scale and Learn

The deliver phase begins with a focused pilot in a representative clinical unit rather than broad rollout. Success measures include medication timing, clinician-reported workload, interruption frequency, and perceived clarity around escalation. Feedback is collected continuously, allowing the intervention to be adjusted as it encounters real-world variability.

Importantly, implementation is treated as the start of learning rather than the endpoint. As staffing patterns change or patient acuity increases, the intervention is revisited and adapted. What remains consistent is the system logic: safe action is made visible, supported, and easier to execute under pressure.

#### Reflection

Across all phases, immediate stabilization actions can occur in parallel with design work. In the example shared, temporary measures, such as manual tracking of time-critical medications or short-term staffing adjustments, may be implemented quickly to reduce risk. These actions are acknowledged as necessary but are also recognized as insufficient. Applying the Double Diamond model allows teams to act decisively in the short term while maintaining focus on longer-term system redesign that reduces reliance on vigilance and heroics.

Incorporating a Double Diamond approach to patient safety problem-solving supports improvement without slowing response or oversimplifying complexity. By separating stabilization from redesign and learning from decision-making, teams can move beyond reactive fixes toward interventions that fit real-world conditions. The model provides a repeatable structure for addressing diverse safety challenges while remaining responsive to the realities of frontline care.

## Beyond the Double Diamond: The AHEAD Framework in Healthcare

While the Double Diamond model offers a useful structure for organizing design work, it is neither the only model available to healthcare teams nor always the most appropriate. Different patient safety challenges demand varying levels of rigor, evidence integration, and adaptive capacity. In settings where interventions must be scientifically defensible, scalable, and responsive to complex clinical conditions, complementary frameworks can provide essential guidance.

In healthcare-specific contexts, the AHEAD framework (Approach to Human-Centered, Evidence-Driven Adaptive Design), developed at Stanford, offers a model explicitly tailored to these demands. AHEAD integrates human-centered design with principles from implementation science, making it particularly well-suited for high-stakes initiatives such as care pathway redesign, digital tool deployment, and system-level safety efforts. The framework emphasizes interdisciplinary collaboration, frontline codesign, and the deliberate integration of empirical evidence throughout the design and evaluation process [11].

### The AHEAD Framework Logic

At its core, AHEAD provides a structured method for applying design thinking in clinical environments where safety, accountability, and scalability are non-negotiable. Unlike design models that emphasize exploration first and evaluation later, AHEAD is explicitly constructed to integrate human-centered inquiry, empirical evidence, and implementation considerations from the outset. This makes it particularly well-suited for patient safety initiatives that must withstand clinical scrutiny, regulatory expectations, and real-world operational constraints [11].

#### Defining the Problem and Assembling the Team

Similar to the Double Diamond, AHEAD begins with deliberate problem definition. The framework emphasizes the importance of articulating a clear, shared understanding of the safety challenge before solutions are proposed. This includes specifying the population affected, the context in which harm occurs, and the outcomes the intervention is intended to influence.

Equally important is the intentional assembly of an interdisciplinary team. AHEAD recognizes that complex safety problems cannot be adequately understood or addressed from a single disciplinary perspective. Effective teams include clinical experts, operational leaders, patients or caregivers where appropriate, and individuals with expertise in design, data, or implementation. The framework explicitly acknowledges that team composition and dynamics influence both the quality of insight generated and the feasibility of resulting interventions [11].

#### Evidence and Inspiration

AHEAD next asks teams to collect information through two streams pursued in parallel: evidence and inspiration. Evidence includes formal sources such as clinical guidelines, utilization data, quality metrics, and published research. Inspiration comes from direct engagement with people and settings. It may include observation, interviews, review of exceptional cases, or examination of practices outside healthcare that illuminate analogous problems.

This dual track matters because healthcare improvement often privileges one type of knowledge at the expense of the other. AHEAD attempts to hold them together. It resists the tendency to design interventions that are evidence-based but poorly fitted to use, or interventions that feel compelling in practice but lack sufficient grounding in what is already known [11].

#### Synthesis and Guiding Principles

Information gathered through evidence and inspiration is then synthesized into a coherent understanding of the system. Rather than producing a list of isolated findings, AHEAD emphasizes the development of guiding principles that articulate how the system should function to support safety. These principles serve as design constraints and decision criteria, shaping subsequent ideation and implementation choices.

In patient safety work, this synthesis phase is particularly critical because safety failures rarely arise from a single cause or isolated breakdown. Instead, they emerge from competing priorities, resource constraints, and misaligned assumptions embedded across clinical, operational, and organizational layers. Synthesis creates the space to surface these tensions explicitly, allowing teams to identify trade-offs that are often invisible in incident reports or performance dashboards. It helps clarify where effort is best applied, which constraints are fixed versus modifiable, and where small changes may exert disproportionate influence on system behavior.

Equally important, synthesis makes assumptions visible and open to challenge. Assumptions about workload, responsibility, risk tolerance, or user capability frequently shape safety interventions but are rarely articulated. Without deliberate synthesis, these assumptions remain embedded in design decisions and can undermine implementation. Structured synthesis methods, such as facilitated sensemaking sessions, affinity clustering, or formal consensus techniques, provide a disciplined way to integrate varied perspectives and reconcile experiential insight with empirical evidence. By doing so, they reduce the risk that design decisions reflect the loudest voices or most familiar narratives rather than a coherent, system-level understanding of the safety problem [11].

### Ideation and Testable Hypotheses

AHEAD approaches ideation with discipline. Rather than treating ideas as creative propositions to be explored informally, potential interventions are explicitly framed as hypotheses about how specific system changes are expected to influence safety outcomes, workflow performance, or user behavior. This hypothesis-driven orientation distinguishes AHEAD from more exploratory design models and aligns ideation directly with implementation science.

In this respect, AHEAD parallels the develop phase of the Double Diamond, where multiple solutions are explored and refined through prototyping. However, AHEAD extends this phase by embedding evaluative intent into the act of prototyping itself. Prototypes are not used solely to assess usability or desirability, but to interrogate safety implications and possible unintended consequences under realistic operating conditions. Each prototype is assessed against the guiding principles established during synthesis, ensuring that concept refinement does not deviate from the safety objectives or evidence base.

Prototyping within AHEAD may take many forms, including workflow simulations, low-fidelity mock designs, environmental walk-throughs, or redesigned communication artifacts. Regardless of form, prototypes are tested in contexts that approximate real clinical conditions, such as time pressure, interruptions, and variable staffing. Feedback is gathered systematically, often combining qualitative observation with quantitative indicators. This disciplined approach allows teams to iterate while remaining aligned with both human-centered insights and evidence-based intent. This reduces the risk that interventions will succeed in a controlled setting but fail when exposed to the complexity of everyday work [11].

### Integrated Evaluation

In AHEAD, evaluation is not deferred until after implementation. It is embedded throughout the design process and continues as interventions are deployed. Evaluation strategies are selected to assess effectiveness, as well as feasibility, fidelity, acceptability, cost, and sustainability. This emphasis reflects the framework's recognition that safety interventions fail as often from poor implementation as from flawed design.

By integrating qualitative and quantitative methods, AHEAD enables teams to detect early signals of success or failure and adapt accordingly. Evaluation thus becomes a mechanism for learning and refinement rather than a retrospective judgment of success [11].

**Reflection**

AHEAD is not a replacement for the Double Diamond. The two frameworks can be used together productively. The Double Diamond offers a clear structure for divergent and convergent work, while AHEAD adds a stronger emphasis on evidence integration, hypothesis-driven development, and ongoing evaluation. In patient safety contexts, that combination can be especially valuable. One framework helps teams see the shape of the design process. The other helps ensure that the intervention remains rigorous, contextually grounded, and evaluable.

## What Design Thinking Is Not

As design thinking gains popularity in healthcare, its terminology is increasingly invoked across strategic plans, quality improvement initiatives, and innovation programs. That growing visibility has also produced confusion. In many settings, design thinking is invoked as a general marker of creativity or modernity rather than as a distinct method. This weakens its usefulness. Clarity requires equal attention to what design thinking does not encompass.

First, design thinking is not just a collection of creative activities. Sticky notes, whiteboards, and ideation games may be visible markers of a design session, but they are not sufficient to constitute a design thinking approach. Without grounding in user research, structured problem framing, and iterative testing, these tools risk becoming performative rather than transformative. As design leaders emphasize, the process must be anchored in purpose, empathy, and system understanding… not just aesthetics or facilitation theater [1].

Second, design thinking is not a substitute for clinical or operational expertise. It complements, rather than replaces, evidence-based medicine, process engineering, and quality improvement (QI). Its strength lies in uncovering insights that other methods may overlook (emotional barriers, behavioral friction, workarounds) and integrating those insights into the design of interventions. In this way, it is a bridge between expert knowledge and lived experience [2].

Third, design thinking is not synonymous with other improvement methods, though it can be used alongside them. Several adjacent frameworks are often confused with or conflated with design thinking, including:

Lean: Originating in manufacturing, Lean focuses on eliminating waste and maximizing efficiency. While it shares design thinking's attention to value creation, Lean emphasizes process optimization, often with less focus on emotional or experiential dimensions [12].

Plan-Do-Study-Act (PDSA): A core method in quality improvement, PDSA cycles encourage small-scale testing of change ideas. However, PDSA typically assumes the problem is already well-defined, whereas design thinking invests time upfront in problem framing through ethnographic research and empathy mapping [13].

Human Factors Engineering (HFE): HFE emphasizes cognitive, physical, and environmental alignment to reduce error and improve system usability. It is highly analytical and often expert-led. Design thinking, by contrast, engages users as codesigners and embraces creativity, even when solutions are not yet technically defined [14].

Each of these frameworks has merit and can be integrated with design thinking when applied thoughtfully. For example, a health system might use design thinking to reframe a challenge (e.g., why patients miss appointments), then apply Lean to streamline the resulting solution (e.g., transportation scheduling), and use PDSA to pilot and refine it over time. The key is discerning which approach is appropriate at each stage of the work. Exploratory design methods are essential for understanding problems and generating options, while implementation-oriented evaluation is required to test, refine, and sustain interventions. Conflating these mindsets risks either premature judgment or unfocused experimentation.

Finally, design thinking is not a shortcut to innovation. It demands time, humility, and patience. It asks teams to slow down before speeding up; to observe, listen, and reframe before acting. When done well, it surfaces insights that can radically shift direction. When done poorly, it risks trivializing human-centeredness into a checkbox.

Understanding what design thinking *is not* is as important as grasping what it *is*. Clarity on this point helps organizations protect the integrity of their design efforts and build trust among those who are asked to participate in the process. Without this distinction, design thinking risks being misapplied as a superficial brainstorming exercise, a one-time innovation workshop, or a substitute for evidence-based improvement. When this happens, frontline staff may experience fatigue or skepticism, particularly if participation does not lead to meaningful change or if creative exploration is followed by abandonment.

Clear boundaries also prevent design thinking from being conflated with traditional project management or rapid solution deployment. Design thinking is not a shortcut around governance or rigor, nor is it a justification for bypassing clinical standards or operational discipline. Instead, it is a structured approach to inquiry and learning that complements, rather than replaces, established improvement and evaluation methods. By articulating what design thinking does and does not encompass, organizations create the conditions for more authentic engagement, more productive collaboration, and more durable impact over time.

## Skills and Mindsets for Practice

While process models and toolkits provide structure, it is the *people* practicing design thinking (and the mindsets they bring) that ultimately determine its success. Unlike methodologies that rely primarily on technical expertise or procedural adherence, design thinking depends on a set of personal and interpersonal capabilities that support curiosity, collaboration, and experimentation. These attributes are increasingly recognized as essential for navigating the complexity and emotional intensity of modern healthcare environments [3].

The first foundational mindset is **curiosity**: a commitment to inquiry over assumption. Design thinkers seek to understand how people experience systems, what adaptations they make, and what gaps exist between intention and impact. This mindset has been shown to enhance problem-sensing skills and reduce premature closure in clinical teams [7]. In nursing education, for example, students trained in design thinking are more likely to identify upstream system failures rather than focusing solely on individual error [4].

A second is *humility*: recognizing that no one person or discipline holds all the answers. In design thinking, clinicians, patients, environmental services workers, and family caregivers are all considered valid sources of insight. This principle stands in contrast to the traditional hierarchy of healthcare knowledge, which often privileges credentialed expertise over lived experience. Teams that model humility create safer spaces for co-creation and shared authorship [7].

*Visual thinking* is another defining feature of design-based work. Healthcare problems are often abstract or entangled in technical language. By translating ideas into journey maps, empathy diagrams, and storyboards, teams externalize their thinking and surface misalignments. These visual tools are particularly effective in interdisciplinary teams, helping diverse stakeholders co-create shared understanding [15].

*Systems awareness* enables design thinkers to view problems not in isolation but as part of interdependent networks. This includes attention to workflows, technologies, policies, cultures, and power structures. Students and clinicians trained in systems thinking are better able to navigate ambiguity, anticipate unintended consequences, and align interventions with broader safety and equity goals [14].

These mindsets are supported by a toolkit of skills and methods that translate well to healthcare improvement. These include:

*Journey mapping* to visualize the patient or provider experience over time

*Personas* to humanize diverse user needs and preferences

*Storyboarding* to map future-state workflows and prototype improvements

*Field observation* to capture contextual insights and environmental constraints

*Low-fidelity prototyping* (e.g., sketches, role-play) to test solutions quickly and iteratively

A 2025 scoping review found that design thinking–based learning approaches, when implemented with hands-on, project-based learning, improved nursing students' confidence in using these tools, especially when the learning was project-based and connected to real healthcare problems [4]. Another study introduced design thinking into a graduate nursing program through interdisciplinary "design sprints" focused on real health system problems. Participants not only developed technical competence with tools like journey maps and service blueprints but also reported increased resilience, adaptability, and leadership confidence [16].

These capabilities should not remain confined to specialized innovation teams. Several health systems have begun integrating design education into leadership development, quality improvement training, and clinical onboarding [17–19]. Doing so increases the likelihood that design methods will become part of everyday improvement work rather than remaining isolated within designated innovation settings.

## Ethical Considerations and Limitations

While design thinking offers powerful tools and mindsets for addressing complex healthcare challenges, its application is not without ethical and practical limitations. As with any method, careless implementation can result in unintended harm, reinforce inequities, or undermine trust. Responsible design practice requires more than creativity; it demands critical reflection, inclusive engagement, and organizational humility.

One of the most pressing ethical concerns is codesign fatigue. Patients, family members, and frontline staff are often asked to participate in workshops, interviews, and feedback sessions without clear follow-up or compensation. When stakeholders share painful experiences or invest time in ideation but see little resulting change, it can breed disillusionment and reduce willingness to engage in future efforts. Recent literature emphasizes the importance of transparency in how insights are used, as well as recognition of contributors' emotional and cognitive labor [20].

A second concern is representation and power dynamics. Design thinking often aspires to inclusivity, but in practice, codesign sessions may exclude marginalized voices: non-English speakers, night-shift workers, disabled individuals, or those with lower digital access. This can lead to solutions that inadvertently reinforce the biases or blind spots of dominant groups. To mitigate this, teams must actively recruit underrepresented perspectives, share decision-making authority, and reflect critically on whose needs are being prioritized [16, 21].

Time and resource constraints also shape ethical use. Design thinking requires deep engagement, iteration, and flexibility. In settings where time is tightly controlled and operational pressure is constant, teams may be tempted to breeze through earlier stages and move directly to ideation or implementation. Projects that skip these critical stages (like ethnographic research or prototyping) to save time may produce shallow results or fail to deliver meaningful improvements. While rapid-cycle design is possible, it must be balanced with methodological integrity [2].

Another limitation is misapplication: using design thinking when it may not be appropriate. Not all problems require human-centered approaches. Issues involving regulatory compliance, infrastructure planning, or acute risk mitigation may be better served by evidence-based protocols or expert consensus. Similarly, not all teams are ready for participatory work. Design thinking requires a baseline of psychological safety, open communication, and leadership support. Without these, the process may surface conflict without resolution or frustrate participants expecting quick fixes [22].

Finally, there is a risk of overstatement. Design thinking is not a silver bullet. It does not guarantee innovation, nor does it replace robust evaluation or policy reform. Some critiques argue that design thinking has been oversold in healthcare settings, used more for branding than substantive transformation. Responsible design practice acknowledges its limitations and complements it with other frameworks, such as implementation science, health equity analysis, and continuous quality improvement [8].

Ethically sound design practice therefore requires explicit attention to scope, representation, power, and follow-through. It also requires enough organizational honesty to recognize when the method is being used well and when it is being used mainly to signal openness or modernity. When practiced with care, design thinking can widen participation and improve system fit. When practiced carelessly, it can deepen fatigue and skepticism.

## Conclusion

Design thinking is useful in patient safety only when it retains methodological discipline. Applied superficially, it becomes little more than a vocabulary of innovation layered onto familiar habits. Applied with care, it changes where inquiry begins, whose experience is treated as evidence, and how quickly organizations move from identifying a problem to settling on a response.

That difference matters most in settings where conventional review captures sequence and deviation more readily than experience. Important parts of harm remain difficult to see unless the investigation can also account for what patients, families, and clinicians were carrying through the event itself. What first appears to be a technical problem may take on a different shape once the emotional, cognitive, and relational dimensions of care are allowed into the analysis.

## References


1. Brown T. Change by design: how design thinking transforms organizations and inspires innovation. Boston: Harvard Business Press; 2009.
2. Ku B, Lupton E. Health design thinking: creating products and services for better health. 2nd ed. Cambridge, MA: MIT Press; 2022.
3. Nursing World. Innovation and design thinking in nursing education and healthcare settings. Online J Issues Nurs. 2025;30(1)
4. Cui Y, Shao Y, Shi H, Qian J, Kang J, Bao K, et al. Emerging trends and hotspots in health monitoring technologies for nursing: a bibliometric analysis. Healthcare Front. 2024;2(3):150–8.
5. Folmer MB, Jangaard K, Buhl H. Design of genuine birth environment: midwives intuitively think in terms of evidence-based design thinking. HERD. 2019;12(2):71–86.
6. Bate P, Robert G. Experience-based design: from redesigning the system around the patient to co-designing services with the patient. Qual Saf Health Care. 2006;15(5):307–10. https://doi.org/10.1136/qshc.2005.016527.
7. Dorst K. Frame innovation: create new thinking by design. Cambridge, MA: MIT Press; 2015.
8. Norman DA. The design of everyday things. Revised and expanded ed. New York, NY: Basic Books; 2013.
9. d.school Institute of Design at Stanford. *Stanford d.school*. Stanford: Stanford University; 2010. Available from: https://web.stanford.edu/~mshanks/MichaelShanks/files/509554.pdf
10. Design Council. The double diamond: a universally accepted depiction of the design process. London: Design Council; 2019.
11. Fischer M, Safaeinili N, Haverfield M, Brown-Johnson C, Zionts D, Zulman D. Approach to human-centered, evidence-driven adaptive design (AHEAD) for health care interventions: a proposed framework. J Gen Intern Med. 2021;36(4):1041–8. https://doi.org/10.1007/s11606-020-06451-4.
12. Graban M. Lean hospitals: improving quality, patient safety, and employee engagement. 3rd ed. Boca Raton: Productivity Press; 2018.

13. Institute for Healthcare Improvement. Science of improvement: testing changes. Boston: IHI. [cited 2026]. Available from: https://www.ihi.org/how-improve-model-improvement-testing-changes
14. Carayon P, Wetterneck TB, Rivera-Rodriguez AJ, Hundt AS, Hoonakker P, Holden R, et al. Human factors systems approach to healthcare quality and patient safety. Appl Ergon. 2014;45(1):14–25.
15. Stickdorn M, Hormess ME, Lawrence A, Schneider J. This is service design doing. Sebastopol: O'Reilly Media; 2018.
16. Holt J, Talsma A, Lloren JI, Eljarrah I, Woehrle L, Avdeev I. Human-centered design in graduate nursing education: outcomes from a cohort study. Nurse Educ. 2025;50(2):68–74.
17. Kaiser Permanente. Garfield Innovation Center. Oakland: Kaiser Permanente. [cited 2026]. Available from: https://about.kaiserpermanente.org/our-story/innovation/garfield-innovation-center
18. Mayo Clinic Center for Innovation. About the Mayo Clinic Center for Innovation. Rochester: Mayo Clinic. [cited 2026]. Available from: https://centerforinnovation.mayo.edu/about/
19. Veterans Health Administration. Veterans health administration experience design. Washington, DC: U.S. Department of Veterans Affairs. [cited 2026]. Available from: https://www.va.gov/experience-design
20. Steen M, Manschot M, De Koning N. Benefits of co-design in service design projects. Int J Des. 2011;5(2):53–60.
21. Bazzano AN, Martin J, Hicks E, Faughnan M, Murphy L. Human-centred design in global health: a scoping review of applications and contexts. PLoS One. 2017;12(11):e0186744. https://doi.org/10.1371/journal.pone.0186744.
22. Liedtka J. Perspective: linking design thinking with innovation outcomes through cognitive bias reduction. J Prod Innov Manag. 2015;32(6):925–38. https://doi.org/10.1111/jpim.12163.

# Humanizing Safety Events 3

## Introduction

Efforts to improve patient safety have traditionally emphasized system reliability, error reduction, and procedural compliance. These aims remain important. They do not fully capture the lived consequences of safety events for the people involved. When something goes wrong in healthcare, whether through a diagnostic delay, a medication error, or a breakdown in coordination, the effects extend beyond physical harm. Patients may experience fear, confusion, betrayal, or grief. Families may lose trust in clinicians and in the institutions expected to protect them. Healthcare professionals may carry guilt, shame, anxiety, or a diminished sense of professional identity.

These experiences are not incidental. They shape how harm is understood, how it is remembered, and whether organizations learn from it in ways that support repair as well as prevention.

The psychological and emotional distress experienced by clinicians involved in adverse events is now widely recognized under the term "second victim syndrome" [1]. Recent studies have shown that clinicians often report acute emotional distress, erosion of professional identity, and longer-term burnout when such events are not followed by meaningful support or reflective debriefing [2–4]. These effects extend beyond individual suffering. They influence retention, team functioning, willingness to


K. Rasmussen, *Rethinking Patient Safety*,
https://doi.org/10.1007/978-3-032-26054-3_3

speak openly, and the wider culture in which safety work takes place.

Even so, many traditional safety investigations remain focused on fact-gathering and policy alignment, with limited room for emotional reflection. Patients and families, meanwhile, are often excluded from the investigative process or included only in ways that do not meaningfully capture their narratives or experiences [5]. That omission can deepen the alienation of those already affected by harm and narrow the organization's opportunity to learn from the event in fuller terms.

Empathy is not a substitute for rigor. It is one of the conditions under which deeper insight becomes possible. When empathy is incorporated into safety investigation, it can bring otherwise obscured dynamics into view: work-arounds performed under strain, unspoken communication failures, hesitation shaped by hierarchy, or gaps in understanding that altered decision-making in real time. It can also create conditions in which clinicians speak more honestly about what happened and what they were carrying through the event, without fear of immediate judgment. For patients and families, more attentive forms of inquiry may offer acknowledgment, validation, and, in some cases, the beginning of repair.

Recent work in human-centered healthcare design and trauma-informed care supports the value of this broader lens. Empathy-driven inquiry has been associated with richer organizational learning, stronger patient and staff engagement, and safer system redesign when patient and clinician experience is treated as a legitimate source of evidence [6, 7].

## Looking Beyond the Clinical Record

When safety events are investigated, clinical documentation often becomes the dominant source of truth. Timelines, medication administration records, communication logs, and progress notes are examined to reconstruct what happened, when it occurred, and which individuals were involved. This documentation is essential for establishing factual sequence and accountability. Yet, by design, it privileges what is measurable and observable over what is felt, perceived, or endured. The clinical record can tell us what occurred, but it rarely captures how the event was experienced by patients, families, or clinicians living through it.

An exclusive reliance on records, checklists, and standardized debrief forms risks flattening complex human experiences into procedural summaries. Emotional distress, moments of uncertainty, hesitation to speak up, and the erosion of trust that often accompany harm are seldom visible in structured documentation. When these dimensions are excluded, safety reviews may overlook critical contextual factors, particularly those related to interpersonal communication, psychological safety, and environmental or workload pressures that shaped decision-making in real time.

Recent literature emphasizes the importance of integrating patient narratives into safety evaluations. For example, the Agency for Healthcare Research and Quality (AHRQ) developed the Consumer Assessment of Healthcare Providers and Systems (CAHPS) Patient Narrative Item Sets, which use open-ended questions to elicit detailed patient stories about their healthcare experiences. These narratives have been shown to uncover aspects of care quality not captured by standard surveys, providing deeper insights into patient-provider interactions and care processes [8].

Empathy-driven methods provide a critical complementary lens. Narrative elicitation techniques, such as open-ended interviews, guided storytelling, or reflective prompts, help surface emotional truths that conventional reviews often miss. These accounts frequently illuminate what safety scientists describe as "soft signals" of system strain: fear of retaliation, intuition dismissed, conflicting priorities, or work-arounds quietly enacted to keep care moving. A 2024 study examining the integration of family voices into incident reviews found that narrative accounts revealed actionable insights into environmental design flaws and communication breakdowns that formal reports had failed to detect [5].

Clinicians themselves may also underreport emotional distress in formal investigative settings. Concerns about blame, professional identity, or reputational harm can suppress honest reflection, particularly in cultures that equate error with individual failure. Trauma-informed design approaches emphasize the need for psychologically safe spaces for sensemaking, using trained facilitators, anonymized narrative tools, and structured emotional debriefs to support clinicians while still enabling system-level learning [7, 9]. Without these supports, the clinical record alone can unintentionally reinforce silence rather than curiosity.

Moving beyond the clinical record does not mean weakening methodological rigor. It means broadening the evidentiary frame. When structured documentation is read alongside lived accounts, healthcare organizations gain a more complete understanding of harm: the procedural sequence of an event, as well as the way it was perceived, interpreted, and carried forward by those involved. That fuller understanding strengthens learning and increases the likelihood that safety work will address not only what failed, but also what made failure harder to see or prevent.

## Methods for Humanizing Safety Reviews

Traditional safety investigations emphasize sequence, deviation, and accountability. Humanizing safety review requires the inclusion of methods that can capture context, experience, and emotional reality with greater precision. These methods do not replace root cause analysis or event reporting systems; rather, they complement them by bringing empathy, subjectivity, and context into focus. By introducing human-centered design artifacts into the investigative process, healthcare teams can illuminate the cognitive, emotional, and environmental factors that shape both harm and healing.

### Personas

Personas are evidence-informed, composite representations of real people affected by a system [10]. In patient safety work, they are neither fictional characters nor simple demographic profiles. Rather, personas are analytical constructs synthesized from interviews, direct observation, chart review, and contextual inquiry to capture recurring patterns in goals, constraints, stressors, motivations, and decision-making behaviors. This approach makes it possible to meaningfully anonymize patients, nurses, physicians, and family members involved in safety events while still preserving the authenticity of their lived experience across groups such as bedside clinicians, patients with chronic illness, caregivers, or trainees navigating competing demands.

Unlike case summaries or incident narratives that anchor analysis to a single event, personas allow teams to reason across time and context. They invite a different line of inquiry, asking what happened, moment to moment, and how a system consistently behaves for someone like this over days, shifts, or care transitions. This distinction is particularly important in patient safety, where harm often arises from cumulative strain, persistent misalignment, or chronic work-arounds rather than from isolated failures.

In practice, personas help counteract hindsight bias and moral judgment by identifying the real constraints under which decisions are made. By making visible factors such as cognitive load, staffing pressures, fragmented information, or emotional fatigue, personas reframe behavior as situated and adaptive rather than negligent. When used in multidisciplinary safety reviews, they serve as a shared reference point that grounds discussion in human reality rather than abstract policy expectations. This technique has been used effectively in simulation and healthcare codesign to foster empathy, alignment, and deeper system insight across diverse user experiences [11] (Fig. 3.1).

## Empathy and Journey Maps

Empathy maps and journey maps are closely related tools within human-centered design, yet they serve distinct analytic purposes in patient safety work. Both are used to surface experience, but they operate at different levels of resolution and over different time horizons. When applied together, they enable safety teams to connect moment-by-moment human experience with the broader system conditions in which harm emerges.

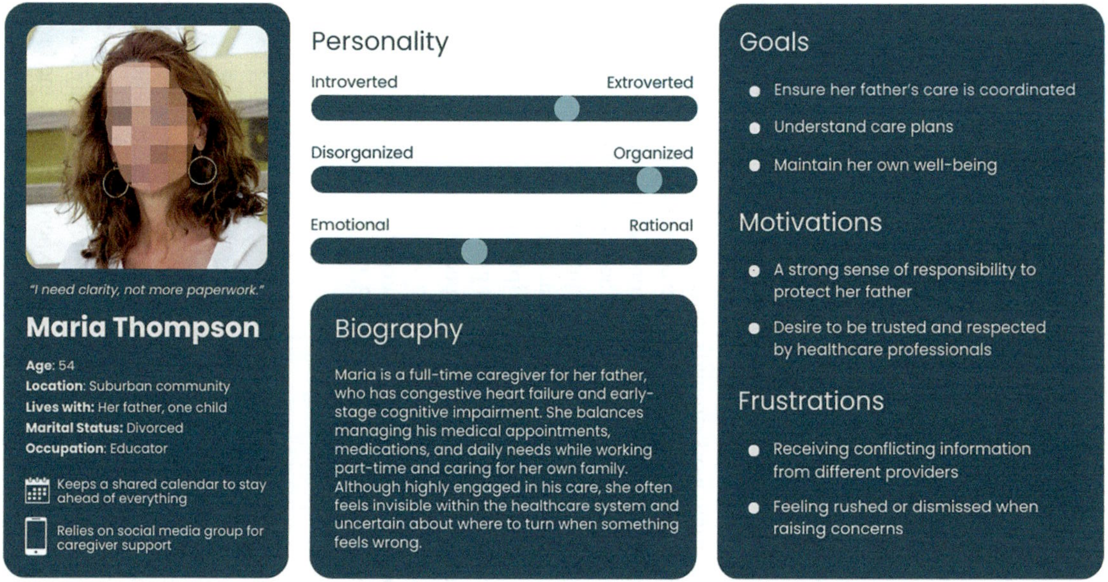


**Fig. 3.1** An example of a composite persona of a patient caregiver used to represent lived experience and contextual constraints in patient safety analysis

Empathy maps focus on internal experience at critical moments. Adapted from service design, they offer a structured way to capture what individuals are thinking, feeling, seeing, hearing, saying, and doing within a specific situation or decision point [12]. In clinical contexts, empathy maps have been used to examine the emotional and cognitive dimensions of care, particularly under conditions of stress, uncertainty, or time pressure [13]. Their value lies in making visible the perceptual and affective states that shape behavior, including fear of escalation, confusion during handoffs, moral distress, or hesitation to challenge authority.

In patient safety investigations, empathy maps help explain why actions that appear irrational or negligent in hindsight were experienced as reasonable or necessary at the time. For example, in a maternal hemorrhage review, the use of empathy mapping revealed that confusion during shift change, combined with the absence of clear visual cues, delayed recognition of patient deterioration despite adherence to documented protocols [14]. By mapping emotional and cognitive load alongside observable actions, investigators gained insight into how system design influenced sensemaking, not just task execution.

Journey maps, by contrast, focus on experience over time across a process or pathway. Patient journey mapping is increasingly recognized in health services research as a structured method for documenting and visualizing how individuals move through complex healthcare systems, including interactions, transitions, barriers, and facilitators encountered along the way. Recent methodological literature defines journey mapping as an approach that captures sequences of touchpoints across the continuum of care, producing visual or narrative representations of how services are actually experienced rather than how they are intended to function [15, 16].

In safety work, journey maps are notably beneficial for identifying where risk accumulates across time, especially at interfaces such as admissions, transfers, handoffs, and discharge. They expose delays, duplications, work-arounds, and breakdowns in coordination that are often invisible when investigations focus narrowly on single events. Experience-based design research has shown that mapping patient journeys can reveal emotional touchpoints, unmet needs, and system fragmentation that directly influence safety and quality outcomes [17, 18]. More recent reviews confirm that journey mapping is increasingly used to understand how people enter, navigate, and exit healthcare systems, highlighting points where system complexity amplifies vulnerability rather than resilience.

Used together, empathy maps and journey maps allow safety teams to move between micro-level human experience and macro-level system flow. Journey maps answer where harm emerges across a pathway; empathy maps explain how it is perceived, interpreted, and responded to at critical moments. This dual perspective is especially important in patient safety, where harm rarely results from a single breakdown but instead arises from the interaction of cumulative system strain and human adaptation. Together, these tools expand safety investigations beyond procedural reconstruction, supporting a more comprehensive understanding of harm as both a system phenomenon and a lived human experience. By integrating experiential insight with process visibility, empathy and journey maps create new opportunities to identify leverage points for redesign that support safer performance under real-world conditions.

## Narrative Elicitation

Narrative elicitation offers a complementary and often underutilized approach to understanding safety events. When storytelling is structured and facilitated within psychologically safe conditions, it allows patients, families, and clinicians to articulate not only what occurred but also how events were interpreted in real time and why particular decisions felt necessary or constrained. These narratives frequently surface contributing factors that remain invisible in formal reviews, including fear of speaking up, unspoken role assumptions, value conflicts, and moral distress. An expanding evidence base suggests that narrative elicitation supports deeper learning from harm, as well as recovery, trust restoration, and collective sensemaking following adverse events [7].

Unlike traditional debriefings or root cause analysis interviews, which are designed to reconstruct timelines and identify deviations from expected processes, narrative elicitation prioritizes meaning-making over fault-finding. Facilitated discussions occur with individuals or small groups and rely on open-ended, non-leading prompts that enable reflection on perception, meaning, and choice, such as:

What were you noticing as the situation developed?
What felt uncertain in that moment?
What options seemed available to you at the time?
What prior experiences or expectations shaped your response?

These conversations are conducted with explicit boundaries that distinguish learning from judgment. Insights are synthesized thematically rather than attributed to individuals, allowing professionals to identify patterns across experiences without reinforcing defensiveness or blame. Additionally, these insights become a foundation for reframing problems, testing assumptions, and identifying opportunities for system redesign.

When applied to patient safety, narrative elicitation broadens traditional event review by adding interpretive depth. Instead of asking whether actions were right or wrong, it reveals how conditions, social dynamics, and cognitive load shaped behavior in real time. In this way, narrative elicitation bridges design thinking and patient safety science, enabling organizations to move beyond procedural explanations toward a richer understanding of how risk and resilience are produced in everyday work.

## Experience-Based Codesign

Experience-based codesign (EBCD) elevates the narrative and empathy-driven methods already discussed by positioning patients, families, and staff as active partners in making sense of harm and shaping solutions. Rather than limiting participation to post-event interviews or feedback collection, EBCD brings stakeholders together to jointly review experiences, identify priorities, and co-create interventions [19]. This approach has been applied across settings, such as oncology, maternity care, and mental health services, particularly in contexts where traditional incident reviews and improvement efforts had failed to produce durable change [20–27]. By grounding redesign efforts in shared experience, EBCD reframes safety events as opportunities for collective learning and repair rather than isolated failures requiring correction [17].

From a design perspective, EBCD shifts the focus from extracting insight to building capability and ownership within the system. It creates structured spaces where experiential knowledge is treated as legitimate evidence alongside clinical data and process metrics. The act of codesign itself becomes an intervention, strengthening relationships, rebuilding trust, and aligning system changes with the realities of care delivery [21].

The use of tools such as narrative elicitation, empathy maps, journey maps, and codesign signals a broader cultural shift in how organizations approach safety. Humanized safety reviews acknowledge that harm is not solely a technical problem to be fixed but a system experience to be understood. By expanding the scope of inquiry beyond procedural failure, these approaches make it possible to see the whole system, not just the point of breakdown, and to embed empathy directly into the architecture of organizational learning.

## Addressing Second Victim Syndrome Through Design

When adverse events occur, the emotional toll extends beyond patients and families. Healthcare professionals, especially those directly involved in the incident, often suffer in silence, experiencing guilt, anxiety, and self-doubt. This phenomenon, known as second victim syndrome (SVS), describes the psychological distress clinicians endure following involvement in patient harm. First described over two decades ago [1], SVS remains a pervasive yet under-addressed consequence of medical error, with recent studies showing that 30% to 60% of healthcare workers report symptoms of SVS at some point in their careers [28].

Despite its prevalence, organizational responses to SVS are often limited or reactive. Traditional incident reviews may inadvertently exacerbate harm by focusing solely on procedural deviations and outcomes, without acknowledging the emotional and moral experiences of those involved. In worst-case scenarios, investigations can feel punitive, reinforcing isolation and fear among staff [29]. This undermines both psychological safety and learning, two cornerstones of resilient safety culture.

Design thinking offers an alternative pathway: one that centers empathy, emotional safety, and co-creation. By integrating trauma-informed principles and user-centered methods, design-led safety reviews can support clinicians as people, not just as actors in a system [7]. This begins with psychological safety: creating structured, facilitated spaces where staff can share their perspectives without fear of blame or repercussion. These conversations emphasize storytelling, reflection, and shared understanding as opposed to judgment.

Personas and empathy maps can also help teams discuss emotionally charged events without centering scrutiny on one identifiable individual. For example, an empathy map based on the recurring experience of a night-shift nurse carrying multiple unstable patients can help a group examine system strain while reducing the defensiveness that often accompanies personal review [6]. These tools preserve emotional truth while creating enough analytic distance to support more open dialogue.

Some institutions have also developed formal peer support programs grounded in human-centered principles. These programs pair affected staff with trained colleagues who can offer empathy, normalization, and guidance in the aftermath of harm. Evidence suggests such interventions both reduce emotional burden and also improve team cohesion and retention [30].

Ultimately, addressing SVS through design means embedding empathy into the fabric of post-event processes, not as an afterthought but as a core component of learning. Organizations that recognize emotional safety as essential to operational safety create the conditions for deeper insights, stronger teams, and more resilient systems.

## Designing Empathy Into Investigation

To humanize safety reviews and support psychological healing, healthcare organizations must adopt methods that surface emotional truths and enable inclusive, reflective inquiry. Empathy-driven investigations emphasize understanding over judgment and context over correction. They rely on practical tools and facilitation techniques that prioritize the emotional safety and lived experiences of both patients and healthcare workers. Several evidence-based methods are emerging as central to this change.

*Emotionally attuned interviews* form the foundation of empathy-based inquiry. This technique prioritizes creating a safe and supportive environment for participants, allowing them to share their experiences without fear of judgment or retraumatization. This approach is particularly effective in trauma-informed forensic interviewing, where understanding and compassion are essential for gathering accurate and comprehensive information [31]. Unlike conventional debriefs that focus on what went wrong, these interviews begin by asking open-ended, nonjudgmental questions: "What were you feeling in that moment?" or "What did you need that you didn't have?" These prompts invite participants to explore not only actions, but perceptions, hesitations, and emotional states. Interviewers trained in trauma-informed communication can recognize distress signals, validate emotional responses, and support constructive reflection without retraumatizing individuals [7].

*Shadowing and contextual immersion* allow investigators and design facilitators to observe systems from the user's perspective [32]. Walking through workflows, experiencing environments firsthand, and witnessing the subtle adaptations staff make in real-time offer insights that rarely surface in written reports. This technique has been used in high-acuity areas such as emergency departments and neonatal care units to uncover communication bottlenecks, spatial constraints, and invisible labor that contribute to safety vulnerabilities [33, 34].

*Collaborative sense-making* brings together multidisciplinary teams, including patients and family members, to jointly analyze incidents. In contrast to siloed reviews, this approach supports shared understanding and reduces cognitive biases by integrating multiple narratives. Techniques such as storytelling circles, empathy mapping, and journey reconstruction allow diverse participants to co-create a timeline of experience, revealing how different roles perceived the same moment in time. These exercises are not only informative; they also build trust and foster mutual respect across professional and experiential boundaries [17].

*Visual storytelling* is also gaining traction in clinical safety contexts. Instead of relying solely on verbal reports or text-heavy timelines, teams use visual tools, such as journey maps, experience timelines, and service blueprints, to externalize and structure events as collective narratives. This fosters emotional accessibility and supports sense-making across diverse team roles. A recent case from Mayo Clinic demonstrated the power of this method: during the setup of a new outpatient clinic amidst the COVID-19 pandemic, service blueprinting was used to visualize patient and staff interactions, highlight operational interdependencies, and surface unseen pain points in the care journey. The visual format helped stakeholders identify priority areas for improvement and build a shared understanding of how individual actions impacted the larger service experience [34]. In patient safety reviews, similar visual methods allow teams to examine the "lived system" rather than just the documented one, bridging the gap between process and perception.

What unites these methods is not sentimentality, but a broader evidentiary view. They allow organizations to investigate how harm was perceived, carried, and produced within the system. That broader view can support more meaningful redesign precisely because it does not reduce safety learning to procedure alone.

## Case Studies: Reframing Through Empathy

Empathy-driven patient safety reviews allow us to reframe adverse events not just as process failures but as deeply human experiences shaped by emotion, environment, and context. The following case studies illustrate this approach, each grounded in published research and expanded through narrative to show how design thinking and empathy tools can illuminate root causes and inform meaningful systems change.

**Case Study 1 Delayed Cancer Diagnosis**
In a study by Koo et al., researchers explored the care journeys of patients undergoing treatment for head and neck cancer. Through in-depth interviews and journey mapping, they uncovered recurring challenges: confusion about follow-up instructions, fear of being dismissed by providers, and barriers to navigating complex care systems, especially among patients with limited health literacy or communication support [35].

To illustrate, consider a synthesized narrative drawn from the study's findings:

> A middle-aged woman, non-native in the healthcare system's dominant language, visited her community clinic repeatedly with nonspecific gastrointestinal symptoms. A fecal occult blood test was eventually ordered and came back positive. However, the result was neither clearly communicated nor followed up in a timely manner. The patient assumed it was not urgent and delayed further care until symptoms worsened. A colonoscopy months later confirmed advanced colorectal cancer.[1]

A traditional review might identify failures in communication, EHR task management, or referral systems. But a narrative-driven investigation, modeled after the study's approach, would surface subtler truths: the patient's hesitation to ask questions, lack of interpreter support, and emotional signals of dismissal. Using empathy maps and communication journey modeling, teams

[1] Based on themes from Koo et al. [35].

could identify friction points—from rushed consultations to poorly explained test results—and codesign new interventions such as visual education tools, navigator roles, and culturally attuned workflows.

In this reframed model, harm is not just a missed follow-up; it is a failure of relational and communicative design.

**Case Study 2 Medication Error**

A widely studied phenomenon in safety literature is the "second victim" experience: when healthcare providers are traumatized by their involvement in harm events. Scott et al. documented how emotional distress, guilt, and fear of blame often follow these incidents, and how systems rarely account for the situational factors influencing decisions in the moment.

Consider a synthesized account reflecting these dynamics:

> A newly returned nurse, still grieving the loss of a family member, floated to an unfamiliar unit during a night shift. She encountered a diabetic patient with a complex regimen and mistakenly administered two overlapping insulin doses. The patient survived, but the incident triggered a root cause analysis focused on documentation and policy adherence.

Through a design-informed debrief process, the nurse's story revealed a more complete picture: unfamiliarity with the unit's layout, absence of a peer double check, and emotional fatigue compounded by grief. An empathy map visualized how stress escalated across the shift. Instead of blame, the response included supportive peer debriefing, environmental redesign of med stations, and pairing float staff with unit-based buddies for orientation.

Rather than isolating the nurse's action as an error, the empathy framework made visible the invisible pressures that shaped it, transforming both support structures and learning culture.[2]

[2]Inspired by second victim research and systems-level stressors [30].

**Case Study 3 Navigating Pediatric Mental Health Care in the ED**

In their 2025 study, Soman et al. explored the barriers to pediatric mental and behavioral health care in emergency departments (EDs) by combining patient journey mapping with provider workflow analysis. The researchers synthesized data from observations, electronic medical records, and staff interviews at four EDs in the southeastern United States. Their findings revealed a complex network of breakdowns in the care experience, particularly during medical and psychiatric evaluations and in the disposition planning phase. These insights provide a valuable foundation for illustrating how systems thinking and empathy-based design can inform safer, more supportive emergency environments [36].

The following narrative is a fictional, synthesized representation of those findings:

> Alex, a 12-year-old child, arrives at a regional ED exhibiting signs of acute anxiety, disorientation, and oppositional behavior. The triage process moves quickly, but due to overcrowding and the limited availability of behavioral health professionals, Alex waits many hours before receiving a formal psychiatric evaluation. The physical environment exacerbates the crisis: bright lighting, noise, and a lack of personal space, amplifying his distress. Staff, although compassionate, appear uncertain and inconsistent in their approach, reflecting their primary training in acute trauma and medical stabilization rather than pediatric behavioral health. Communication with external services to coordinate follow-up care proves slow and fragmented, further delaying transfer to a specialized treatment center.[3]

These challenges are not isolated; they are symptomatic of deeper systemic issues. The researchers identified that many EDs lack tailored protocols for pediatric mental and behavioral health patients, resulting in inconsistent workflows and care fragmentation. Moreover, physical design limitations, such as the absence of quiet rooms or sensory-safe spaces, contribute to escalated distress and increased risk. Staff expressed both a desire and a need

[3]Based on themes from Soman et al. [36].

for more structured support and training when managing these vulnerable cases.

To address the barriers identified in the study, the research team proposed a series of design and workflow interventions aimed at improving the quality and responsiveness of care for pediatric mental and behavioral health patients in emergency departments. These included developing integrated care protocols that standardize how ED teams assess and manage pediatric MBH cases, thereby reducing variability and improving coordination. Environmental modifications were also emphasized, such as creating quiet, sensory-friendly spaces within the ED to minimize stress for patients in crisis. Additionally, the study stressed the importance of specialized training programs to equip emergency staff with the skills and confidence needed to navigate the unique complexities of pediatric behavioral emergencies. Finally, the researchers advocated for improved communication systems between EDs and external mental health services, ensuring more timely transfers and continuity of care. Together, these interventions reflect an empathy-informed approach to redesigning pediatric emergency care environments [36].

These case studies illustrate how empathy-centered methods, such as journey mapping, narrative inquiry, and contextual analysis, can reveal deeper systemic contributors to harm than traditional reviews typically capture. By foregrounding lived experience and situational context, they shift the focus from compliance and correction to understanding and co-creation. Regardless of the setting or challenge, these examples demonstrate that patient safety is not merely a function of protocols but of how well systems are designed to support real people in real conditions. The following section builds on these insights by translating them into actionable design strategies that move from reflection to implementation.

## From Insight to Practice

Empathy-based review is valuable only if the insight it generates changes how systems are designed. The practical challenge is to move from reflection to action without losing the human complexity that made the insight meaningful in the first place.

Design thinking offers one pathway because it provides methods for translating experience into intervention. Once empathy maps, journey maps, and narratives have clarified where burden, confusion, or relational breakdown is occurring, those patterns can be reframed into focused design questions. Prompts—such as "How might we make discharge communication easier to understand under stress?" or "How might we reduce emotional isolation for staff after harm events?"—help shift the work from description toward response [37].

Low-fidelity prototyping is especially useful at this stage. In healthcare, a prototype may be as simple as a revised conversation script, a mock-up of a new communication tool, a redesigned family update process, or a structured peer-support workflow. The purpose is not polished. It is to make a response tangible enough to test before institutionalizing it. Ku and Lupton describe this kind of prototyping as a key bridge between human-centered insight and actionable redesign [6].

Testing should not be limited to the outcome alone. Early evaluation should examine whether an intervention is understandable, usable, and emotionally credible for those expected to engage with it. In design-oriented safety work, this often means collecting direct feedback from staff, patients, and families as the intervention is refined. Mikkelsen and colleagues, for example, showed how participatory design in medication transition planning allowed teams to revise tools iteratively in response to real user experience [38].

Meaningful implementation also depends on organizational support. Teams need protected time, leadership sponsorship, and the ability to revise interventions as they encounter real use. Innovation centers and embedded design functions within systems such as Kaiser Permanente, Mayo Clinic, and the Veterans

Health Administration illustrate one way organizations have begun to support this infrastructure [39–41]. Their importance lies not merely in the existence of specialized teams, but in the signal that human-centered redesign is part of institutional work rather than an extracurricular activity.

The final challenge is evaluative. Organizations often measure harm outcomes without attending sufficiently to changes in trust, burden, clarity, or perceived safety. Yet, these experiential dimensions are often the earliest signs that a redesign is functioning well or failing quietly. Robert and colleagues have shown that the long-term sustainability of improvement depends on both the technical outcome and on whether staff and patients experience the change as meaningful and workable [42].

Moving from insight to practice is therefore not a matter of attaching an action plan to a narrative. It requires a different standard of translation: one in which emotional and relational evidence remains part of the redesign process rather than being discarded once implementation begins.

## Conclusion

Humanizing safety review adds more than narrative depth to an existing process. It changes what becomes visible in the event itself. Once fear, uncertainty, burden, and adaptation enter the analysis, the problem often no longer appears to be only a lapse in compliance or execution. It begins to look more like a mismatch between what the system required and what the people within it could reasonably absorb, interpret, or manage in real time.

That shift matters because it changes what counts as a meaningful explanation, which forms of evidence are treated as relevant, and where redesign ought to begin. An investigation tied too narrowly to procedural deviation may miss the conditions that made the event more likely and more difficult to interrupt. A fuller account does not weaken rigor. It places rigor in closer contact with the realities of care.

When the human experience of harm is taken seriously, safety inquiry becomes less concerned with producing a neat retrospective account and more concerned with asking what the event reveals about the system that produced it.

## References

1. Wu AW. Medical error: the second victim. The doctor who makes the mistake needs help too. BMJ. 2000;320(7237):726–7. https://doi.org/10.1136/bmj.320.7237.726.
2. Quillivan RR, Burlison JD, Browne EK, Scott SD, Hoffman JM. Patient safety culture and the second victim phenomenon: connecting culture to staff distress in nurses. Jt Comm J Qual Patient Saf. 2016;42(8):377–86. https://doi.org/10.1016/S1553-7250(16)42053-2.
3. Potter HA, O'Brien-Irr MS, Henninger MW, Flanagan-Priore C, Winkelstein P, Harris LM. Association between second victim syndrome and burnout among physicians at a single center. J Vasc Surg. 2023;77(3):897–904. https://doi.org/10.1016/j.jvs.2022.08.060.
4. Busche IM, Moretti F, Purgato M, Barbui C, Wu AW, Rimondini M. Psychological and psychosomatic symptoms of second victims of adverse events: a systematic review and meta-analysis. J Patient Saf. 2020;16(2):e61–74. https://doi.org/10.1097/PTS.0000000000000589.
5. Dukhanin V, Dy SM, Sharma R, Vass M, Zhang A, Bass EB, et al. Patient and family engagement in patient safety practices: a making healthcare safer rapid response review. J Patient Saf Risk Manag. 2024;29(3):135–47. https://doi.org/10.1177/25160435241234332.
6. Ku B, Lupton E. Health design thinking: creating products and services for better health. 2nd ed. Cambridge, MA: MIT Press; 2022.
7. Goldstein E, Chokshi B, Melendez-Torres GJ, Rios A, Jelley M, Lewis-O'Connor A. Effectiveness of trauma-informed care implementation in health care settings: systematic review of reviews and realist synthesis. Perm J. 2024;28(1):135–50. https://doi.org/10.7812/TPP/23.071.
8. Agency for Healthcare Research and Quality. CAHPS patient narrative item sets. Rockville: AHRQ; 2023. Available from: https://www.ahrq.gov/cahps/surveys-guidance/item-sets/elicitation/index.html
9. Ahmed Z, Ellahham S, Soomro M, Shams S, Latif K. Exploring the impact of compassion and leadership on patient safety and quality in healthcare systems: a narrative review. BMJ Open Qual. 2024;13(Suppl 2):e002651. https://doi.org/10.1136/bmjoq-2023-002651.
10. Miaskiewicz T, Kozar KA. Personas and user-centered design: how can personas benefit product design processes? Des Stud. 2011;32(5):417–30. https://doi.org/10.1016/j.destud.2011.03.003.
11. Dominello A, Cheek C, Clay-Williams R. The use of personas to involve consumers in healthcare co-design: a scoping review. BMC Health Serv Res. 2025;25:142. https://doi.org/10.1186/s12913-025-10847-6.

12. Hampshire N, Califano G, Spinks D. Empathy mapping. In: Mastering collaboration in a product team. Cham: Apress; 2022. p. 101–18. https://doi.org/10.1007/978-1-4842-8291-7_6.
13. Thompson C, Barforoshi S, Kell C, Banerjee D. Uncovering the patient experience: empathy mapping promotes patient-centered care for improved heart failure patient outcomes. J Card Fail. 2016;22(8):587–8.
14. Sherman JP, Hedli LC, Kristensen-Cabrera AI, Lipman SS, Schwandt D, Lee HC, et al. Understanding the heterogeneity of labor and delivery units: using design thinking to assess environmental factors that contribute to safety in childbirth. Am J Perinatol. 2020;37(6):638–46.
15. Bulto LN. Patient journey mapping: emerging methods for mapping patient experiences and interactions in healthcare systems. Eur J Cardiovasc Nurs. 2024;23(4):429–37.
16. Davies EL, et al. Reporting and conducting patient journey mapping research: a scoping review. BMJ Open. 2022;12(5):e057815.
17. Bate P, Robert G. Experience-based design: from redesigning the system around the patient to co-designing services with the patient. Qual Saf Health Care. 2006;15(5):307–10. https://doi.org/10.1136/qshc.2005.016527.
18. Locock L, Boaz A. Drawing straight lines along blurred boundaries: qualitative research, patient and public involvement in medical research. BMJ Open. 2019;9(11):e031310.
19. Wiig S, Storm M, Aase K, Gjestsen MT, Solheim M, Harthug S, et al. Investigating the use of patient involvement and patient experience in quality improvement in Norway: rhetoric or reality? BMC Health Serv Res. 2013;13(1):206.
20. Cooper K, Gillmore C, Hogg L. Experience-based co-design in an adult psychological therapies service. J Ment Health. 2016;25(4):293–8.
21. Donetto S, Tsianakas V, Robert G. Using experience-based co-design (EBCD) to improve the quality of healthcare: mapping where we are now and establishing future directions. London: King's College London; 2014.
22. Graber N, Canova N, Bryant-Lukosius D, Robert G, Navarro-Rodrigo B, Trueb L, et al. Reflections on the opportunities and challenges of applying experience-based co-design (EBCD) to phase 1 clinical trials in oncology. Health Expect. 2024;27(4):e14068.
23. Hawke LD, Sheikhan NY, Bastidas-Bilbao H, Rodak T. Experience-based co-design of mental health services and interventions: a scoping review. SSM Ment Health. 2024;5:100309.
24. NHS England. Co-production: a literature review and guide. London: NHS England; 2023. Available from: https://www.england.nhs.uk/wp-content/uploads/2023/03/B1498_ii_Co-production-a-literature-review.pdf
25. Palmer VJ, Weavell W, Callander R, Piper D, Richard L, Maher L, et al. The participatory zeitgeist: an explanatory theoretical model of change in

an era of coproduction and codesign in healthcare improvement. Med Humanit. 2019;45(3):247–57.
26. Piper D, Iedema R, Gray J, Verna R, Holmes L, Manning N. Utilizing experience-based co-design to improve the experience of patients accessing emergency departments in new South Wales public hospitals: an evaluation study. Health Serv Manag Res. 2012;25:162–72.
27. Ream E, Tsianakas V, Verity R, Oakley C, Murrells T, Robert G, et al. Enhancing the role of carers in the outpatient chemotherapy setting: a participatory action research project. London: King's College London; 2013.
28. Seys D, Panella M, Russotto S, Strametz R, Mira JJ, Van Wilder A, et al. In search of an international multidimensional action plan for second victim support: a narrative review. BMC Health Serv Res. 2023;23:816. https://doi.org/10.1186/s12913-023-09816-2.
29. Strametz R, Mira JJ, Sousa P. The second victim phenomenon: comprehensive support and systemic change in healthcare. Int J Qual Health Care. 2024;36(3):mzad108. https://doi.org/10.1093/intqhc/mzad108.
30. Scott SD, Hirschinger LE, Cox KR, McCoig M, Brandt J, Hall LW. The natural history of recovery for the healthcare provider "second victim" after adverse patient events. BMJ Qual Saf. 2009;18(5):325–30. https://doi.org/10.1136/qshc.2009.032870.
31. Lee M. Trauma-informed forensic interviewing: creating safety through compassion. Huntsville: National Child Advocacy Center; 2023. Available from: https://www.ncacia.org/post/trauma-informed-forensic-interviewing-creating-safety-through-compassion
32. Goodrich J, Ridge D, Cartwright T. A qualitative study exploring patient shadowing as a method to improve patient-centred care: ten principles for a new gold standard. Int J Qual Health Care. 2022;34(2):mzac016.
33. Sarver WL, Seabold K, Kline M. Shadowing to improve teamwork and communication: a potential strategy for surge staffing. Nurse Lead. 2020;18(6):597–603. https://doi.org/10.1016/j.mnl.2020.08.004.
34. Bartch VM, Vetting Wolf TL, Lee SA, Poncelet SA, Nemec SL, Morgenthaler TI. A service blueprint approach to prioritize operational improvements in a new outpatient clinic. Health J Deliv Sci Innov. 2023;11(4):100126. https://doi.org/10.1016/j.hjdsi.2023.100126.
35. Koo Y, Kim E, Jo Y, Nam I. Patient experience factors and implications for improvement based on the treatment journey of patients with head and neck cancer. Cancers (Basel). 2023;15(8):2263. https://doi.org/10.3390/cancers15082263.
36. Soman DA, Koscelny SN, Neyens D, Dietrich A, Narasimhan M, Taaffe K, et al. Using patient journey mapping and provider workflows to understand process barriers to pediatric mental and behavioral health care in emergency departments. Appl Ergon. 2025;126:104189. https://doi.org/10.1016/j.apergo.2024.104189.

37. Brown T, Wyatt B. Design thinking for social innovation. Stanford Soc Innov Rev. 2010;8(1):30–5.
38. Mikkelsen TH, Søndergaard J, Kjær NK, Nielsen JB, Ryg J, Kjeldsen LJ, et al. Designing a tool ensuring older patients the right medication at the right time after discharge from hospital: the first step in a participatory design process. BMC Health Serv Res. 2024;24(1):211. https://doi.org/10.1186/s12913-024-10621-4.
39. Kaiser Permanente. Garfield Innovation Center. Oakland: Kaiser Permanente. [cited 2026]. Available from: https://about.kaiserpermanente.org/our-story/innovation/garfield-innovation-center
40. Mayo Clinic Center for Innovation. About the mayo clinic center for innovation. Rochester: Mayo Clinic. [cited 2026]. Available from: https://centerforinnovation.mayo.edu/about/
41. Veterans Health Administration. Veterans health administration experience design. Washington, DC: U.S. Department of Veterans Affairs. [cited 2026]. Available from: https://www.va.gov/experience-design
42. Robert G, Sarre S, Maben J, Griffiths P, Chable R. Exploring the sustainability of quality improvement interventions in healthcare organisations: a multiple methods study of the 10-year impact of the "productive Ward: releasing time to care" programme in English acute hospitals. BMJ Qual Saf. 2020;29(1):31–40.

# Reframing: From Problems to Possibilities

# 4

## Introduction

In healthcare, the way a safety problem is defined exerts considerable influence over everything that follows. The problem statement guides what is examined, which stakeholders are consulted, which forms of evidence are treated as legitimate, and which interventions come to appear appropriate. For that reason, framing is not a preliminary step of minor importance. It is one of the most consequential acts in patient safety work.

Many improvement efforts begin with a problem statement that is too narrow, too technical, or too shaped by institutional habit. A fall may be framed as noncompliance with protocol. A delay in care may be described as a scheduling inefficiency. A medication error may be treated as inattentiveness. These formulations can be convenient because they are legible within organizational systems of measurement and accountability. They are often also incomplete.

Reframing is the practice of revisiting those initial formulations and asking whether the problem has been defined at the right level, from the right vantage point, and with sufficient regard for context. Within design thinking, reframing is one of the central means by which a problem space is opened rather than prematurely closed. It allows teams to shift perspective, reexamine assumptions, and consider alternative definitions of success.


K. Rasmussen, *Rethinking Patient Safety*,
https://doi.org/10.1007/978-3-032-26054-3_4

The difference this makes can be substantial. Consider the difference between asking, "How do we reduce discharge delays?" and "How might we help patients feel ready and confident to go home?" The first question may lead to interventions focused on bed management or discharge timing protocols. The second might uncover gaps in patient education, trust, or caregiver coordination. Both are valid, but only one invites a more holistic view of the system and its human participants.

Reframing requires more than creativity. It demands curiosity, humility, and a willingness to suspend early certainty. These qualities are not always rewarded in healthcare environments that are structured around urgency, risk control, and efficiency. Yet as patient safety challenges grow in complexity, linear thinking is no longer sufficient. Systems thinking has taught us that events often emerge from dynamic, interacting factors rather than single causes. Design reframing takes this further by helping teams explore what the problem really is before jumping to fix it.

The value of reframing lies in its effect on what becomes thinkable. It does not solve the problem by itself. It changes the conditions under which a more adequate response can be developed.

## Common Framing Traps in Healthcare Safety

In patient safety work, the way a problem is initially framed often sets the outer limits of what becomes visible, discussable, and actionable. Problem statements are intended to bring clarity. They also carry assumptions. These assumptions may concern causality, responsibility, severity, scope, or which features of the situation matter most. When they remain unexamined, they can narrow the space of inquiry before the work has properly begun. Recognizing common framing traps is therefore not an exercise in abstraction. It is a way of identifying where safety work may become constrained by its own starting language.

## Linear Causality Bias

Healthcare safety has long been influenced by linear cause-and-effect logic: identify the error, locate its root cause, and apply a corrective action. This approach has provided valuable structure and accountability, particularly in settings where reliability is essential. Yet in complex clinical environments, where care unfolds across time, roles, technologies, and shifting conditions, linear explanations often prove insufficient.

When harm is framed as the result of a single failure, such as a missed handoff or an incomplete order, attention is drawn toward isolated moments rather than the broader system and the layers of dynamics that shaped them. This framing can obscure how risks accumulate, how risk adaptations interact, and how trade-offs are made under pressure. It reinforces retrospective bias in investigations [1]. Reframing away from linear causality does not reject rigor; it expands it. It allows safety work to move from asking "What failed?" to asking "What conditions made this outcome more likely?" and, in doing so, opens the door to more meaningful system-level insight.

## Symptom-Focused Framing

Many patient safety initiatives concentrate on visible symptoms rather than the conditions that produce them. Problems are frequently defined by what is most readily measured, such as missed appointments, delays, errors, or nonadherence. When an issue is framed narrowly, for example, as "reducing no-show rates," proposed solutions often gravitate toward expedient fixes like automated reminders or enforcement mechanisms. While these interventions may offer short-term improvement, they tend to address only the most observable expression of the problem.

Symptoms, however, function as signals within a system. They indicate friction, unmet needs, or misalignment between how care is designed and how it is experienced. In the case of missed appointments, underlying contributors may include transportation barriers, scheduling inflexibility, competing life demands, or erosion of trust between patients and the healthcare system. Lydon's examination of root cause analysis in non-healthcare industries cautions that addressing symptoms without interrogating deeper causality can obscure fundamental drivers of failure and, in some cases, introduce new risks or unintended consequences [2].

When teams pause to reframe symptom-focused challenges, the problem space often expands to include logistical, relational, and experiential dimensions that were previously overlooked. This change moves patient safety work beyond reactive correction toward exploratory learning, creating opportunities to design interventions that address root conditions rather than repeatedly treating their visible manifestations.

## Metric-Centered Framing

Performance metrics play an essential role in healthcare safety, supporting accountability, benchmarking, and regulatory oversight. Yet when metrics become the primary or exclusive lens through which safety problems are defined, they can inadvertently narrow inquiry and constrain learning. Problems framed predominantly around scores, thresholds, or penalties tend to generate solutions optimized for measurement rather than for meaning, experience, or long-term resilience.

For example, an organization focused on reducing readmission rates may frame the problem as one of discharge efficiency or care coordination compliance. This framing often leads to interventions aimed at accelerating discharge processes or standardizing follow-up workflows. While such actions may improve reported performance, they can overlook broader contributors to readmission risk, including patient understanding, caregiver capacity, social support, and trust in the care plan. When metrics dictate framing, improvement efforts risk prioritizing what is most visible to reporting systems rather than what most strongly shapes safety and outcomes [3].

Reframing beyond metrics does not diminish their value; it restores their role as signals rather than endpoints. When teams treat performance data as prompts for deeper inquiry, rather than definitive problem statements, they create space to ask more generative questions: What does this metric represent in lived experience? What conditions make improvement difficult or fragile? What success might look like beyond the number itself? In this way, metrics become gateways to understanding, supporting safety interventions that are compliant, context-sensitive, human-centered, and more likely to endure.

## Exclusion of Emotional and Relational Dimensions

Many patient safety challenges are framed in technical terms that fail to capture the emotional and relational dynamics at play. For example, communication breakdowns are often interpreted as failures in information transfer…something to be corrected with scripts, checklists, or revised workflows. But this framing misses the human drivers of miscommunication, such as mistrust, fear, emotional fatigue, or misaligned expectations between clinicians and teams.

Research on psychological safety, particularly the work of Edmondson and others, shows that team members are far more likely to speak up, report errors, and adapt effectively when they feel emotionally safe to express concerns without fear of reprisal [4]. Without this foundation of trust, even well-intentioned protocols can falter in high-stakes environments. In healthcare, the emotional labor of caregiving, the vulnerability of patients, and the asymmetries of authority and expertise all shape how information is shared…or withheld.

When safety problems are framed solely around procedural compliance, we risk designing interventions that address behaviors while ignoring the environments that produce them. In contrast, reframing through the lens of psychological safety and emotional design invites us to ask different questions: *Why didn't someone feel safe speaking up? What structural or cultural signals discouraged vulnerability? How might we create conditions that foster relational trust?*

By recognizing emotional safety as a core design parameter, teams can develop more effective and sustainable solutions: ones that focus not just on reducing risk but on creating cultures of openness, mutual respect, and collective accountability.

## Role-Centric Framing

Safety challenges are often defined from the viewpoint of a single role or group, typically those responsible for oversight, regulation, or clinical decision-making. While these perspectives are critical, they rarely capture the full experience of care. Patients, family caregivers, and other roles frequently encounter risks, workarounds, and ambiguities that remain invisible to formal structures. Role-centric framing limits who is seen as a legitimate contributor to problem definition and solution design.

A recent systematic review of patient and caregiver involvement in chronic kidney disease research found that increased engagement resulted in improved recruitment, richer contextual insights, and more relevant deliverables [5]. This finding supports long-standing evidence from person-centered care literature, which emphasizes that healthcare is most effective when patient values, autonomy, and relational dynamics are honored [6]. By failing to include those voices early in problem definition, healthcare organizations risk creating solutions that are technically sound but miss critical dimensions of safety: emotional, cultural, and experiential.

Reframing through a role-inclusive lens intentionally expands the boundary of inquiry: How does this problem appear to someone receiving care? To someone coordinating across shifts? To someone balancing competing priorities at the bedside? By asking these questions, teams can uncover misaligned assumptions, unaddressed needs, and new opportunities for shared ownership of both the problem and its resolution. This inclusive framing enhances both the design integrity and the sustainability of patient safety solutions.

## From Constraints to Possibilities

Taken together, these framing traps reveal how easily safety work can become constrained by its own assumptions. Linear causality, symptom fixation, metric dominance, emotional detachment, and role-based blind spots each narrow the field of inquiry in different ways, yet they often coexist in the same investigation. Each of these framing traps represents a moment where inquiry narrows prematurely. Left unexamined, they can lead to solutions that are technically sound yet contextually misaligned, efficient yet fragile.

By learning to recognize how problems are framed, healthcare teams gain greater freedom to question assumptions, surface hidden dynamics, and imagine alternatives that better reflect the complexity and humanity of care. This lays the groundwork for reframing not as a rhetorical exercise but as a disciplined, learnable skill, one that strengthens both the quality and the impact of patient safety work.

## Reframing as a Design Skill

Reframing is sometimes treated as a matter of instinct or creativity, as though certain people simply see problems differently. In practice, reframing functions more usefully as a disciplined skill. It can be learned, strengthened, and applied systematically within patient safety work.

At its core, reframing involves a shift in perspective. That shift may occur by redefining who the problem is for, by broadening the system boundary under consideration, by changing the unit of analysis, or by altering the criterion of success. Within design practice, reframing often changes the intervention only because it first changes what the team understands the problem to be [7].

Several distinct forms of reframing are especially relevant in healthcare.

*User-centered reframing* redirects attention from institutional priorities (such as throughput or compliance) to the lived experiences of those receiving and delivering care (such as readiness, dignity, or trust). Robert and Cornwell's work on Experience-Based Co-Design (EBCD) is a foundational example of this change. By engaging patients and staff in co-design sessions grounded in real narratives, their approach reframes safety and quality challenges from "Where did the process break down?" to "What caused confusion, fear, or dignity loss during the care experience?" [8]. This lens helps surface relational and emotional needs that are often invisible in data-driven reviews, grounding improvement efforts in the realities of end users.

*Context-sensitive reframing* challenges one-size-fits-all thinking by grounding problems in the specific dynamics of each care environment. A process that works well in a high-resource surgical unit may fall apart in a rural emergency department or behavioral health setting, not because the goal is flawed, but because the surrounding conditions are different. Staffing, layout, technology access, and cultural norms all shape how safety issues appear and what solutions are viable. Informed by systems and design theory, this approach calls on teams to see the system as it actually is, not as they assume it to be [9].

*Possibility-oriented reframing* moves the conversation away from control and deficiency toward opportunity. Drawing from public sector innovation theory, this approach encourages teams to question current limitations and explore "what if" scenarios that reveal untapped opportunities. Rather than starting with what is broken, this lens begins with what might be possible, opening space for new partnerships, alternative models, and inclusive co-creation. It shifts safety work from reactive fixes to proactive transformation [10].

These forms of reframing do not reduce rigor. They alter where rigor is applied. Instead of assuming the problem statement is already stable, teams treat it as provisional and worthy of examination. Several internal dispositions support this work:

*Curiosity*, the willingness to hold off on early conclusions and explore multiple interpretations of a problem. In design, curiosity is not just a personality trait; it is a disciplined practice supported by tools and methods. Techniques such as contextual inquiry, shadowing, and journey mapping help teams uncover patterns that would otherwise remain hidden. These methods support open-ended exploration and create space for insights to emerge before solutions are defined [11].

*Humility*, or the ability to recognize the limits of one's own perspective and invite others into the frame. In innovation theory, humility is essential to co-creation. Rather than asserting control, it encourages leaders and teams to shift into inquiry and make room for the lived experience of patients, families, and frontline workers to reshape how problems are understood. Humility builds psychological safety, reduces blind spots, and improves the quality of reframing [10].

*Systems literacy*, or the ability to understand how outcomes result from the interactions between people, technologies, environments, and policies. Hollnagel's work on Safety-I and Safety-II emphasizes that safety is not the absence of failure but the presence of system conditions that support adaptation and success. Systems literacy helps teams identify how interdependencies shape performance and how small changes in one area can produce unexpected effects elsewhere [1].

These capacities matter because patient safety problems are rarely solved well by superficial reformulation. Reframing requires teams to look again at what they think they know, what they are taking for granted, and what kinds of change they have made difficult to imagine by the way the issue has initially been named.

It also helps address initiative fatigue. When frontline staff are invited only to comment on already-defined solutions, improvement work can feel imposed. When they are invited into the work of framing the problem itself, participation becomes more substantive. That often improves both the quality of insight and the likelihood of later adoption.

The next section turns from these conceptual capacities to the practical methods that support reframing in day-to-day safety work.

## Methods and Tools for Reframing

While design-based methods are increasingly visible in healthcare innovation and experience work, they remain underused in routine patient safety practice. Most safety teams rely on linear analytical tools that clarify process breakdowns but struggle to surface social, emotional, and contextual contributors to harm. Design methods complement these approaches by expanding how problems are defined before solutions are selected.

The tools introduced below are drawn from human-centered design, design thinking, and systems innovation practice. They are intentionally adaptable and can be used independently or in combination across safety huddles, interdisciplinary improvement efforts, and organization-wide initiatives. Rather than replacing established safety methods, they extend them by shifting attention upstream, inviting teams to slow down just enough to see differently and explore safety challenges with greater curiosity, openness, and shared understanding before moving to action.

### How Might We (HMW) Questions

Originally developed and popularized by the design firm IDEO, the "How Might We" method converts insights and observations into possibility-focused prompts [12]. Rather than framing problems around failure or blame, HMW questions reframe challenges in ways that encourage inclusive exploration. For example, instead of asking, "Why do nurses skip hand hygiene?" a reframed HMW question might be, "How might we make hand hygiene easier to perform in moments of time pressure?" The language intentionally signals openness to multiple solutions and focuses attention on opportunity rather than deficit.

## Insight Clustering

Insight clustering is a qualitative synthesis method that helps teams make sense of large volumes of observational or interview data. Team members write down individual quotes, behaviors, or insights on sticky notes or digital cards and group them based on similarity. This visual clustering process reveals emergent themes that may be overlooked in linear or quantitative analyses. It supports shared understanding across diverse roles and disciplines and helps surface emotional, environmental, and systemic patterns that contribute to safety challenges. When used in post-incident reviews or proactive design research, it can uncover friction points in the user experience and provide a foundation for reframing safety problems more inclusively and meaningfully [11].

## Reframing Matrix

A reframing matrix is a structured tool that helps teams examine a problem from multiple vantage points. One axis typically represents different stakeholder groups, such as patients, nurses, physicians, or caregivers, while the other captures categories like emotional experience, workflow constraints, information gaps, or environmental factors. By systematically populating this grid, teams can identify blind spots, surface tensions, and recognize where assumptions may be misaligned across roles. This approach is especially valuable in complex systems where safety challenges are shaped by overlapping responsibilities, competing priorities, and diverse interpretations of the same event. The matrix encourages inclusive problem definition and helps ensure that the framing of the issue reflects the lived experiences of those most affected [13].

## Story Reframing

Story reframing is a method that invites teams to revisit a safety incident or process breakdown by intentionally shifting the point of view. Instead of analyzing the event solely through clinical documentation or formal review, teams re-express the situation from a different perspective—such as that of the patient, a family member, or a non-clinical team member. This narrative shift helps reveal emotional cues, cognitive demands, or contextual factors that may be overlooked in traditional evaluations. By broadening the narrative lens, teams can move beyond procedural breakdowns and identify deeper contributors to harm, including unmet human needs, environmental stressors, or communication mismatches. When paired with tools like journey maps or personas, story reframing supports a more holistic, empathetic understanding of safety challenges [14].

## Reframing in Action: What It Could Look Like

Reframing is a powerful skill for addressing real-world challenges in patient safety. When reframing becomes a routine part of work rather than a one-time exercise, organizations strengthen their capacity to design interventions that reflect how care is actually delivered and experienced. This approach acknowledges variability not as a failure to control, but as a defining feature of complex systems. It creates space to consider competing priorities, emotional labor, environmental constraints, and the adaptations people make to keep care moving forward. Over time, this deeper understanding supports improvements that are more resilient, context-sensitive, and aligned with human capability.

### Reframing Vignettes

The following scenarios are intentionally hypothetical. Their purpose is not to model best practice, but to illustrate how reframing changes the trajectory of inquiry and the nature of resulting interventions.

### Reframing "Reducing Discharge Delays" as "Design Clarity for Discharge Readiness"

In a typical hospital setting, delays in patient discharge are often framed as a throughput problem. The language around the issue is operational: discharges must be expedited, beds turned over faster, barriers removed. This framing leads to interventions like discharge checklists, escalation policies, or reminders in electronic medical records, all of which may streamline documentation but fail to address the root cause of confusion around readiness.

Now imagine a team instead chooses to frame the issue as: "How might we design shared clarity around discharge readiness?" This reframing shifts the focus from moving people out to aligning around what "ready" truly means—for the patient, the family, and the care team. In this hypothetical scenario, the team explores how different disciplines interpret readiness and discovers that while physicians often base decisions on medical stability, patients and nurses highlight emotional preparedness, home support, and functional needs. This insight leads the team to co-create a digital discharge readiness view that includes patient-defined goals, expected date ranges, and real-time updates across care roles. The new framing not only reduces confusion and last-minute delays but also improves patient confidence and continuity of care at home.

### Reframing "Nonadherence" as "Supporting Decision Confidence in Complex Regimens"

Medication nonadherence is frequently framed in terms of patient compliance: patients are expected to follow instructions, and when they don't, it's seen as a deviation to correct. This framing places responsibility primarily on the individual and often prompts solutions like automated refill reminders, alerts, or repeated counseling.

But what if the problem were reframed as: "How might we support decision confidence in the face of complex treatment regimens?" This lens focuses on the decision-making journey itself.

In a hypothetical primary care setting, a multidisciplinary team conducts empathy interviews with patients managing multiple chronic conditions. They find that patients are not resisting care but navigating trade-offs between side effects, affordability, work demands, and mental load. Reframing the issue helps the team shift its approach from education-based "fixes" to relational solutions, such as codeveloped care timelines, simplified medication packaging, and routine check-ins to revisit goals of care. The intervention becomes not just about adherence, but about building capacity for informed, confident decisions over time.

#### Reframing "Preventing Patient Aggression" as "Designing Safe Engagement Environments"

In inpatient behavioral health units, staff safety is an ongoing concern. Patient aggression is often framed as a behavioral risk to be controlled. Interventions tend to focus on surveillance, restraint protocols, or de-escalation training. While important, these approaches often reinforce an adversarial dynamic and overlook the environmental and relational conditions that shape behavior.

Consider instead a reframed challenge: "How might we design environments that promote safe, respectful engagement?" In this hypothetical example, a unit-based team explores patient-staff interactions, physical space design, and the structure of daily routines. They discover that sensory overload, unfamiliar staff rotations, and lack of personal agency contribute to patient distress. Through collaborative design sessions with staff and individuals with lived experience, they imagine small environmental changes, such as predictable schedules, softer lighting, and co-created safety plans, that promote calm, connection, and trust. The result is not a behavioral management plan, but an environment that reduces the likelihood of escalation by design.

## Leadership and Cultural Implications

Reframing is a team-level practice. It also has implications for leadership and organizational culture. Leaders influence safety work not simply by approving resources or setting targets, but by shaping how problems are named and what kinds of inquiry are treated as legitimate.

When a leader frames a safety issue as a compliance failure, the range of likely responses narrows toward reinforcement, monitoring, and enforcement. When the same issue is framed in terms of trust, communication burden, or system fit, a different set of questions becomes available. Framing is therefore not neutral. It directs attention, legitimizes certain forms of evidence, and makes some solutions seem more reasonable than others [7].

One of the most effective ways leaders can embed reframing into organizational life is by normalizing it in existing structures. Safety event reviews, team huddles, and quality meetings all provide natural opportunities to pause and ask: "Are we solving the right problem?" or "What might we be missing from another perspective?" These questions don't require new resources, just the cultural permission to step back before moving forward.

When reframing is built into improvement routines, it becomes a lever for deeper engagement. Staff are more likely to feel ownership when invited to describe how problems are experienced… not just how they should be fixed. Such inclusivity can reveal blind spots in how problems have historically been defined, especially when those definitions exclude particular roles, identities, or patient experiences. The result is solutions that are more equitable, sustainable, and context sensitive.

However, shifting toward this way of working requires cultural support. Many healthcare organizations, especially those under financial or regulatory pressure, default to predictability and speed. But reframing introduces a different tempo: one that values reflection before resolution. Psychological safety becomes essential here: people need to feel safe to voice uncertainty, share dissenting views, or challenge dominant narratives [4].

Leadership behaviors make the difference. Asking open-ended questions, allocating time for generative inquiry, and celebrating learning (not just outcomes) signals that reframing is not just accepted but valued. As Bason notes in public sector innovation, institutions that embrace ambiguity and invite co-creation are better equipped to tackle complex, persistent challenges [10]. In safety work, this means empowering teams to challenge assumptions and design solutions that are not just reactive but transformative.

Importantly, reframing is not a solo activity. It's most powerful when done collectively, across disciplines and roles. Teams often operate with different mental models, shaped by their training, responsibilities, or proximity to the issue. Without structured opportunities to explore how each group frames a problem, important insights can go unspoken. Tools like insight clustering, reframing matrices, and story reframing help make thinking visible and turn distributed knowledge into an aligned direction.

Yet even when supported, reframing may face resistance. Teams may perceive it as inefficient or misaligned with established workflows. These perceptions deserve attention, but they can also be reframed. Rather than being viewed as an extra step, reframing should be positioned as a quality safeguard: one that reduces wasted effort, aligns interventions with actual needs, and prevents solutions that solve the wrong problem.

Over time, organizations that cultivate this habit build stronger problem-solving muscles. Teams begin to anticipate misalignments earlier, stakeholders feel more connected to the process, and solutions land with greater relevance and clarity. Leaders who spotlight moments when reframing made a difference reinforce the value of the practice and help embed it into the organization's identity.

Reframing is not about replacing what works. It is about expanding what's possible. In complex care systems, where safety emerges not just from protocols but from how people think, collaborate, and respond to uncertainty, reframing is both a discipline and a cultural differentiator.

## Conclusion

Reframing alters patient safety work at an early but consequential point. It shifts attention away from the first available explanation and toward a more deliberate examination of what kind of problem is actually present, who is experiencing it, and which system conditions are shaping it. That movement can seem modest. In practice, it often changes the entire direction of the response.

Its value lies in more than producing a more inventive way of describing the problem. It can prevent organizations from acting too quickly on formulations that are tidy, familiar, and incomplete. Once a problem has been narrowed too soon, improvement efforts often become efficient responses to the wrong level of difficulty. Reframing interrupts that pattern. It keeps inquiry open long enough for hidden assumptions, excluded perspectives, and deeper structural conditions to become visible.

The quality of any intervention depends in part on the quality of the problem definition that precedes it. When framing remains shallow, the resulting solution may be well executed yet still fragile. When framing becomes more precise, a wider range of responses comes into view, including responses that are better aligned with the realities of care. The next difficulty is not how to describe the problem more elegantly but how to generate responses that are genuinely worth testing.

## References

1. Hollnagel E. Safety-I and safety-II: the past and future of safety management. Farnham: Ashgate; 2014.
2. Behrhorst J, Gale B, Manaoat C. The evolution of root cause analysis. PSNet perspective. Rockville: Agency for Healthcare Research and Quality; 2025. Available from: https://psnet.ahrq.gov/perspective/evolution-root-cause-analysis
3. Lipsitz LA. Understanding health care as a complex system: the foundation for unintended consequences. JAMA. 2012;308(3):243–4. https://doi.org/10.1001/jama.2012.7551.
4. Edmondson AC, Bransby DP. Psychological safety comes of age: observed themes in an established literature. Annu Rev Organ Psychol Organ Behav. 2023;10:55–78. https://doi.org/10.1146/annurev-orgpsych-120920-055217.
5. Gutman T, Coghlan D, Craig J, Guha C, Jaure A, Jesudason S, et al. Systematic review of patient and caregiver involvement in CKD research. Kidney Int Rep. 2025;10(6):1657–72. https://doi.org/10.1016/j.ekir.2025.03.012.
6. Grover S, Fitzpatrick A, Azim F, Ariza-Vega P, Bellwood P, Burns J, et al. Defining and implementing patient-centered care: an umbrella review.

Patient Educ Couns. 2022;105(7):1679–88. https://doi.org/10.1016/j.pec.2021.12.022.
7. Brown T. Change by design: how design thinking transforms organizations and inspires innovation. Boston: Harvard Business Press; 2009.
8. Robert G, Cornwell J, Locock L, Purushotham A, Sturmey G, Gager M. Patients and staff as co-designers of healthcare services. BMJ. 2015;350:g7714. https://doi.org/10.1136/bmj.g7714.
9. Kolko J. Wicked problems: problems worth solving. Austin: Austin Center for Design; 2012.
10. Bason C. Leading public sector innovation: co-creating for a better society. 2nd ed. Bristol: Bristol University Press; 2018.
11. Hanington B, Martin B. Universal methods of design: expanded and revised (125 ways to research complex problems, develop innovative ideas, and design effective solutions). Beverly: Rockport Publishers; 2019.
12. Kelley T, Kelley D. Creative confidence: unleashing the creative potential within us all. New York: Crown Business; 2013.
13. Morgan M. Creating workforce innovation: turning individual creativity into organisational innovation. St Leonards: Allen & Unwin; 1993.
14. Bate P, Robert G. Experience-based design: from redesigning the system around the patient to co-designing services with the patient. Qual Saf Health Care. 2006;15(5):307–10. https://doi.org/10.1136/qshc.2005.016527.

# From Insight to Ideation in Patient Safety

# 5

## Introduction

Once a patient safety problem has been framed more carefully, another difficulty appears. Insight does not automatically produce a useful response. Teams may arrive at a more accurate understanding of the problem and still default to the same categories of intervention they would have selected earlier: additional training, policy reinforcement, new reminders, or tighter monitoring. In many healthcare settings, that movement happens quickly. The space between recognizing a problem and settling on a solution is often far narrower than the complexity of the situation warrants.

This narrowing is understandable. Clinical environments are structured around accountability, operational constraint, and pressure to act. Under those conditions, familiar responses can feel safer than exploratory ones. They are easier to explain, easier to authorize, and easier to align with institutional routines. The difficulty is that they may also leave the underlying source of the problem largely undisturbed. A system may be reframed with greater accuracy and still produce an intervention shaped more by organizational habit than by what the reframing has actually revealed.

Ideation becomes important at that point. Its function is not to introduce creativity for its own sake or to suspend practical judgment indefinitely. It creates a disciplined interval in which more



K. Rasmussen, *Rethinking Patient Safety*,
https://doi.org/10.1007/978-3-032-26054-3_5

than one response can be generated before the field narrows again. In patient safety work, that interval matters because the first plausible solution is not always the most useful one, and the most institutionally familiar solution may not be the one most closely aligned with the problem as now understood.

Research on collective problem-solving and organizational creativity has shown that groups often converge too early, especially when hierarchy, evaluation pressure, and time constraint shape how ideas are generated and received [1–3]. Healthcare teams are especially vulnerable to this pattern. They work in settings where reputational risk is visible, expertise is stratified, and speaking provisionally may feel costly. Under those conditions, idea generation requires more structure than conventional brainstorming typically provides.

The issue, then, is not whether patient safety teams are capable of generating ideas. They are. The more important question is how idea generation can be structured so that it expands the range of responses rather than simply reproducing the most available ones.

## The Principles of Effective Ideation

The term *brainstorming* is frequently used in quality and process improvement work as a shorthand for collaborative idea generation. However, a substantial body of research in social and cognitive psychology suggests that traditional interactive brainstorming, especially verbal, real-time group ideation, often yields fewer ideas than approaches that begin with individual idea generation and then pool contributions. This pattern is commonly attributed to production blocking, evaluation apprehension, and social loafing, which can reduce both idea fluency and originality in group settings [4–8].

These limitations become more pronounced in hierarchical, high-accountability environments such as healthcare. Status differentials and professional identities may influence whose ideas are voiced or adopted within teams. In clinical settings where reputational risk and professional credibility are highly visible, individuals may be less willing to offer speculative ideas or dissenting perspectives, particularly when topics are sensitive or emotionally charged [9]. As a result, traditional brainstorming sessions may inadvertently reinforce existing power gradients, producing incremental rather than transformative ideas.

Design-based ideation methods offer a more structured alternative that can better support psychological safety and broader participation. These approaches do not depend on verbal spontaneity or extroverted confidence. Instead, they use structure to separate divergence from evaluation, reduce avoidable social bias, and create protected space for quieter or lower-status voices to contribute. In doing so, they tend to expand the range of ideas generated and improve the likelihood that selected concepts are attentive to user needs and contextual constraints, which is foundational for feasibility and equity in implementation [10, 11].

Four principles differentiate effective ideation from conventional brainstorming in patient safety work.

## Structured Divergence and Convergence

Creative problem-solving is not a single event but a patterned rhythm. Divergence expands the option space by encouraging the generation of multiple possibilities without immediate filtering. Convergence synthesizes, prioritizes, and refines those possibilities in actionable directions. When these stages are collapsed, as they often can be with informal brainstorming, creative fluency declines because participants attempt to generate and evaluate simultaneously [5].

Experimental evidence demonstrates that premature evaluation reduces originality and overall ideational output [4, 6]. By deliberately separating divergent and convergent phases, facilitators create protected cognitive space for exploration before introducing constraint. In patient safety contexts, this distinction is particularly important. Without it, teams may default quickly to familiar interventions (i.e., checklists, reminders, additional training) rather than exploring broader system redesign.

## Psychological Safety as a Precondition for Idea Fluency

Ideation requires interpersonal risk-taking. Participants must be willing to propose incomplete, unconventional, or uncertain ideas. Psychological safety (the shared belief that it is safe to take interpersonal risks within a team) is associated with greater willingness to speak up, question assumptions, and contribute novel suggestions, all of which are foundational to idea generation in teams [9].

In environments where reputational risk is highly visible, such as healthcare patient safety, evaluation apprehension can suppress creative contribution [5]. Structured techniques such as brainwriting and silent idea generation reduce production blocking and decouple contribution from immediate social judgment, resulting in greater idea volume and diversity [7, 12]. These methods do not merely increase participation; they reshape *who* participates and *how*.

## Sequencing Creativity and Judgement

One of the most common mistakes in group ideation is evaluating ideas while they are still being generated. In safety-focused environments, where risk mitigation and compliance are central, the impulse to evaluate can be strong and immediate. Early critique can narrow the space of exploration and reduce idea fluency. When participants anticipate judgment in real time, they are more likely to self-censor, default to familiar options, or withhold unconventional suggestions [4].

Research in social and organizational psychology helps explain why. During idea generation, individuals are particularly vulnerable to evaluation apprehension and status dynamics. Production blocking and self-monitoring consume cognitive bandwidth that would otherwise support associative thinking and novelty. Experimental studies have repeatedly shown that separating idea generation from evaluation increases both the quantity and diversity of ideas produced, particularly in complex problem domains [5, 13, 14].

That said, the goal of design-based ideation is not to eliminate critique altogether. Evidence from innovation and team research suggests that well-timed, task-focused dissent can improve idea quality and decision outcomes when psychological safety is present [9, 15]. Constructive debate helps surface assumptions, test feasibility, and refine promising directions. The key variable is sequencing [13, 14].

Effective ideation therefore separates divergence from convergence. During divergence, teams suspend evaluation to protect fluency and cognitive risk-taking. During convergence, they deliberately reintroduce structured critique, using agreed-upon criteria to assess feasibility, impact, equity, and system fit. This temporal separation allows creativity and rigor to operate in partnership rather than in competition.

In patient safety work, this distinction is especially important. Regulatory pressure, reputational risk, and accountability structures make early evaluation almost reflexive. Without intentional facilitation, critique can arrive before ideas have fully formed. When teams instead make evaluation a deliberate second act, they create conditions where bold thinking can emerge and disciplined refinement can follow.

## Constructive Constraints as Catalysts for Innovation

While divergence expands possibility, too much ambiguity can feel overwhelming or unfocused. Well-framed constraints can enhance originality by channeling creative effort [16]. Constraints focus attention, reduce cognitive overload, and sharpen problem-solving energy.

In patient safety work, constraints might include time frames ("testable within 30 days"), resource boundaries ("no additional staffing"), or scope limitations ("pilot on one unit"). Design scholarship emphasizes that innovation often emerges not despite constraints, but because of them [10, 11]. When thoughtfully framed, constraints move teams from abstract imagination to implementable experimentation.

Together, these four principles provide a psychologically informed framework for ideation in patient safety. The practical implication is clear: effective idea generation is not the product of an unstructured brainstorm but of intentionally designing the conditions and sequencing that allow teams to expand possibilities before narrowing toward action.

## Tools and Techniques for Ideation in Patient Safety

The challenge in patient safety work is rarely that teams lack concern or commitment. More often, the problem lies in the absence of deliberate mechanisms for expanding the range of possible responses before convergence begins. In clinical environments, idea generation is often informal, time-compressed, and shaped by professional hierarchy. Structured ideation methods are useful because they interrupt this pattern and create a disciplined route into broader possibility.

The methods discussed below are not detached from the realities of healthcare work. They are intended for use in safety huddles, event review follow-up, redesign sessions, and quality improvement forums. Their function is not to produce novelty for its own sake, but to help teams consider interventions that better reflect the complexity of the systems they are trying to improve.

### Brainwriting

Brainwriting is a written, low-pressure method of idea generation that reduces production blocking and evaluation apprehension. Rather than speaking ideas aloud in real time, participants generate ideas individually in writing for a defined interval, then pass their ideas to another participant who builds upon or modifies them in subsequent rounds.

This structure accomplishes several things simultaneously:

- It separates idea generation from social performance.
- It reduces status influence.
- It increases idea volume.
- It supports cognitive incubation between rounds.

Research comparing interactive brainstorming with written or nominal techniques demonstrates that independent idea generation followed by aggregation yields higher idea fluency and often greater originality than real-time verbal ideation [5, 6, 17].

In patient safety contexts, brainwriting is particularly useful when:

- The topic is sensitive (i.e., precursor event, workflow breakdown).
- Hierarchy may inhibit contribution.
- The team is interdisciplinary.
- Time is limited, but participation must be broad.

## How to Facilitate Brainwriting in a Patient Safety Setting

A typical brainwriting session can be conducted in 20–30 min and requires only paper (or a shared digital board), writing utensils, and a clearly framed prompt.

1. *Frame the challenge clearly.* Begin with a focused, possibility-oriented question, such as: "How might we reduce near misses during medication handoffs?" Emphasize that this is a divergent phase. No evaluation will occur during idea generation.
2. *Set time boundaries.* Provide 3–5 min for participants to silently write as many ideas as possible on their paper. Encourage volume over polish.
3. *Rotate and build.* At the end of the round, have participants pass their sheet (or digital column) to another person. The next participant adds new ideas or builds on existing ones. Repeat for 2–4 rounds.

4. *Cluster and synthesize.* After the final round, collect the ideas, group similar concepts, and move deliberately into a convergence phase using predefined criteria such as feasibility or impact.
5. *Close the loop.* Provide visibility regarding what will happen next. Even a brief summary of the top themes reinforces psychological safety and signals that all contributions matter.

When facilitated with clear boundaries and disciplined convergence, brainwriting shifts ideation from performative contribution to equitable participation. It allows patient safety teams to generate a breadth of options quickly while minimizing hierarchy, production blocking, and premature critique [12].

## Role-Storming

Role-storming builds on traditional ideation by inviting participants to generate ideas while temporarily adopting a different perspective. Instead of responding as themselves, individuals ideate from the standpoint of a defined role, such as a patient, a family caregiver, a new graduate nurse, a night-shift pharmacist, or even a future version of the organization. This technique draws on cognitive distancing: when individuals speak "as" someone else, they are more likely to suspend self-censorship and professional defensiveness. By shifting focus to the role instead of the person, role-storming loosens habitual patterns of reasoning, unlocking more expansive thinking [18, 19].

Participants may assume roles such as:

- A newly diagnosed patient
- A night-shift nurse
- A brand-new medical resident
- A family caregiver with limited English proficiency

In patient safety work, where professional identity and hierarchy strongly shape discourse, perspective shifting serves an additional function. It temporarily decouples ideas from personal ownership. When a participant speaks "as a caregiver" or "as a novice clinician," the idea becomes exploratory rather than declarative. This can reduce evaluation apprehension and lower defensiveness, both of which are known to suppress idea generation in group settings [5].

In patient safety work, role-storming is particularly useful when:

- Solutions appear stuck in operational language.
- Stakeholder misalignment is evident.
- Teams struggle to integrate patient or caregiver perspectives.
- Hierarchical dynamics constrain contribution.

### How to Facilitate Role-Storming in a Patient Safety Setting

1. *Select the roles or personas.* Roles can be drawn from previously constructed personas or journey maps created during reframing work, recent safety event narratives, or representative stakeholder groups.
2. *Frame the prompt.* Formulate the problem or challenge into an ideation prompt for participants, such as a How Might We statement. For example, "*How might we create a peaceful environment on a telemetry unit?*" Instruct participants to respond only as their assigned role or persona with ideas.
3. *Generate ideas in rounds.* Facilitate this brainstorming in short, timed intervals (e.g., 5 min per round). Consider having participants rotate roles after each round. Encourage them to speak as the persona.
4. *Synthesize emerging patterns.* After divergence, encourage participants to identify conflicting priorities across roles, unmet emotional needs, and opportunities for alignment.

Healthcare safety failures can frequently arise from misaligned mental models across roles. What appears efficient from an administrative perspective may feel rushed from a clinician's standpoint. What seems clinically complete may feel confusing to a family member. Role-storming does not assume empathy; it operationalizes perspective-taking within the ideation process.

The method also aligns with research on perspective-taking and creativity, which suggests that deliberate viewpoint shifts can increase idea novelty and reduce fixation on initial solution paths [5]. In interdisciplinary teams, structured perspective exercises have been associated with broader solution sets and improved integrative thinking [10].

Importantly, role-storming is not theatrical improvisation; it is a cognitive tool. The aim is not performance but reframing through the embodiment of alternate system positions. When integrated into safety improvement work, role-storming strengthens the recognition of relational dynamics, helps teams anticipate unintended consequences, and focuses ideation efforts across all stakeholder needs.

## Reverse Brainstorming

Most ideation methods ask teams to generate solutions directly. Reverse brainstorming intentionally inverts that logic. Instead of asking how to solve a problem, participants are first asked how to guarantee its failure. This structured inversion draws from traditions of lateral thinking and cognitive reframing, which suggest that disrupting habitual problem frames can loosen entrenched assumptions and expand the solution space [18, 19].

In patient safety, this method can be especially potent. Safety problems often carry emotional weight, professional sensitivity, and implicit defensiveness. Directly asking, "How do we fix this?" may produce socially desirable answers or incremental refinements. By contrast, asking, "How could we ensure this fails every time?" introduces psychological distance. That distance allows participants to articulate uncomfortable truths in a way that feels safe: without direct accusation.

Cognitive research on creative problem-solving indicates that exposure to contrasting or oppositional framings can reduce fixation and increase idea novelty [5]. Inversion interrupts linear cause-effect reasoning and makes hidden norms visible. It surfaces vulnerabilities that may be normalized within a system but are rarely named explicitly.

In healthcare, this structured reversal can create permission to identify latent risk factors without attaching blame to individuals. The focus shifts from "who failed?" to "what conditions would reliably produce failure?"

### How to Facilitate Reverse Brainstorming in a Patient Safety Setting

1. *Invert the question.* Format the problem to be solved or the challenge into a question, then reverse the question. For example, if the original challenge is "How might we improve handoff reliability?" the inverse question for ideation would be "How might we guarantee failed handoffs every time?"
2. *Intentionally encourage divergence.* Have participants generate as many "failure strategies" as possible. Examples might include increase interruptions during handoff, eliminate all safety checks, assume critical information is obvious, etc.
3. *Synthesize all ideas.* Help the group identify any recurring themes with their failure strategies, such as ambiguous ownership, information fragmentation, etc.
4. *Invert the ideas again.* Leverage each failure strategy and/or theme as a design opportunity. For example, if an identified theme is ambiguous ownership, come up with as many ideas as possible on how to ensure explicit ownership. This second inversion transforms latent vulnerabilities into actionable interventions.

By expanding the problem space in an unexpected direction, reverse brainstorming complements more traditional ideation tools. It does not replace root cause analysis or risk assessment but rather provides a human-centered lens for exploring how harm emerges when systems are left misaligned, misunderstood, and/or mismanaged.

However, this technique must be facilitated with care, especially in emotionally charged settings or when safety events have resulted in harm. The goal is not to mock or trivialize serious issues but to use cognitive inversion as a tool for deeper system insight. When introduced with clear boundaries and psychological safety, reverse brainstorming can help teams see risks more clearly and respond more creatively.

Reverse brainstorming reflects a foundational insight from design practice: generative thinking improves when participants are temporarily released from the pressure to be right. By suspending the expectation of immediate correctness, teams can examine system vulnerabilities more candidly and with less defensiveness. This orientation is consistent with systems-based approaches to safety, which emphasize how conditions, interactions, and constraints shape behavior over time rather than locating failure in isolated acts [10]. By articulating credible pathways to breakdown in advance, teams strengthen anticipatory capacity rather than relying solely on retrospective correction. In high-stakes clinical environments, this disciplined inversion provides a structured way to surface fragility early, before it turns into harm.

## SCAMPER

SCAMPER is a systematic ideation technique that prompts teams to intentionally alter existing processes rather than attempt wholesale reinvention. The acronym represents seven cognitive moves: Substitute, Combine, Adapt, Modify, Put to another use, Eliminate, and Rearrange [20]. Each prompt directs attention to a specific dimension of change, helping teams interrogate assumptions embedded in current workflows [10].

In healthcare safety, many problems are not caused by a complete absence of structure, but by structures that have ossified. Processes evolve incrementally, adapt locally, and become normalized over time. SCAMPER is useful in these contexts because it does not require teams to imagine a blank slate. Instead, it asks them to examine what already exists and consider how it might be intentionally varied.

Rather than offering abstract prompts, SCAMPER provides a disciplined sequence of modification lenses. It does not demand novelty for its own sake; it demands deliberate inspection of how the current system is constructed.

For example, consider a recurring issue: increased patient falls during shift change. Instead of asking, "How do we prevent falls during handoff?" a team using SCAMPER might explore:

- *Substitute*: What element of the current handoff could be replaced? Could a verbal-only report be substituted with a brief bedside mobility check?
- *Combine*: Could the shift report be combined with a structured safety sweep for high-risk patients?
- *Adapt*: Are there practices from intensive care or perioperative environments that manage transitional vulnerability more effectively?
- *Modify*: Could the timing, duration, or sequencing of handoff be adjusted to reduce unattended intervals?
- *Put to another use*: Could an existing rounding checklist be repurposed to include fall-risk confirmation during transition?
- *Eliminate*: What nonessential activities occurring during shift change increase environmental complexity?
- *Rearrange*: Could the order of handoff report prioritize high-fall-risk patients first rather than following room order?

This reorients the conversation from compliance monitoring ("Are we following the protocol?") to structural design inquiry ("How is this moment configured, and how might it be configured differently?").

Healthcare organizations operate under constant constraints: staffing limits, regulatory oversight, budget pressure, reputational risk, and time scarcity. Open-ended ideation can sometimes feel impractical. SCAMPER's strength is that it operates within constraint. It directs modification within the existing system. It is therefore well-suited for:

- Post-event reviews where teams feel stuck
- Redesigning entrenched workflows
- Incremental improvement of safety communication tools
- Situations where feasibility must remain visible

### How to Facilitate SCAMPER in a Patient Safety Setting

SCAMPER is effective when used to examine a specific safety-relevant process rather than a vague or abstract challenge. In patient safety work, it is particularly useful after a patient safety opportunity has been identified and has clear contributing factors, but no solutions have been selected. The goal is not to generate creative novelty for its own sake, but to deliberately interrogate how the current system is structured.

1. *Define the safety target clearly*. Begin with a narrowly defined process or vulnerability (e.g., "medication reconciliation during admission").
2. *Establish psychological ground rules*. Reinforce with participants that this is a design exercise, not a performance review. Make explicit that the focus is on modifying system conditions rather than evaluating individual behavior. This protects psychological safety and keeps the session forward-looking.
3. *Select relevant SCAMPER prompts*. This tool does not require all seven prompts to be used. Choose two to four that align with the safety issue. For example, for a documentation-related challenge, "Eliminate" and "Modify" might surface more insights.
4. *Time exploration*. Allocate 5–7 min per prompt. Ask participants to generate ideas silently first, then share. This reduces anchoring and allows quieter voices to contribute. Capture ideas visibly without critique.
5. *Surface assumptions*. After generating ideas for each prompt, ask the group: "What does this reveal about how the current process is designed? What risks are built into the way this is currently structured?" This step connects ideation back to systems thinking and prevents the session from devolving into superficial tweaks.

6. *Transition to convergence*. Once all selected prompts have been explored, the team can shift into evaluation, assessing ideas against feasibility, safety impact, testability, etc.

When facilitated in this way, SCAMPER becomes more than a creativity exercise; it becomes a structured mechanism for redesigning risk. By intentionally varying existing system components, patient safety teams can expose hidden fragilities and generate targeted, testable interventions without defaulting to compliance-only responses.

Together, these ideation tools provide disciplined mechanisms for expanding the solution space before narrowing it. They do not rely on charisma, artistic talent, or unstructured creativity. Instead, they offer structured ways to interrupt habitual thinking, reduce hierarchy-driven distortion, and generate options that are both imaginative and testable. When embedded into daily safety huddles, post-event reviews, and improvement collaboratives, these methods signal a shift: idea generation becomes a designed process rather than an informal exchange.

Yet even the most thoughtfully selected tool cannot compensate for a climate that suppresses contribution. Structured methods create opportunity. The surrounding conditions determine whether that opportunity is realized.

## Creating the Conditions for Creativity in Healthcare Teams

Even the most carefully chosen ideation method is unlikely to produce useful results if the surrounding conditions suppress contribution. In healthcare, this issue is significant. Clinical teams operate under strong time pressure, visible hierarchy, and high accountability. Under such conditions, creativity does not emerge spontaneously. It depends on an environment in which it becomes possible to think aloud without immediate reputational cost.

Take the physical setting. A room set in rows with a lectern at the front might reinforce hierarchy and prompt guarded thinking. In contrast, a flexible space with movable chairs, flip chart papers scattered across walls, and objects that provoke reflection, such as faux patient artifacts or journey maps, signals a different kind of engagement. These subtle design choices can shift energy from compliance to curiosity.

But true creativity emerges only when people believe they can speak up without judgment or reprisal. Extensive healthcare research shows that psychological safety—believing it is safe to take interpersonal risks—is vital to enabling learning, collaboration, and yes, innovation within clinical teams [21, 22]. In a psychologically safe unit, a new nurse can raise concerns about a process, not because they are perfect, but because the team has decided that putting ideas forward is more important than protecting one's facade.

Patient safety teams and leaders reinforce this through language, modeling inquiry, and encouraging imperfect ideas. Statements like "tell me what surprised you" or "let's learn from that, not judge it" create cultural space for learning and experimentation. These cues, even more than formal rules, signal to teams that ideation is valued, not just tolerated.

Creativity in healthcare also requires balancing structure with freedom. Too much structure makes ideation feel rigid; too little risks drift. Well-integrated design tools provide just enough scaffolding to guide thought, then promptly release it. Novel prompts like SCAMPER or timed silence followed by a group share (in brainwriting), provide anchor points for exploring possibilities without suffocating them.

Considering power dynamics and diversity is equally important. In multidisciplinary teams (especially where power imbalances exist), hierarchy can mute important perspectives. Introverts and newer team members are all too familiar with the instinct to defer. Design choices like round-robin sharing, anonymous input options, or seating that mixes disciplines intentionally invite more voices into the dialogue. These aren't procedural niceties; they're problem-solving accelerants.

Diversity in teams offers potential but requires inclusion to unlock creative value. Research in organizational collaboration shows that diverse teams generate more novel solutions when inclusive norms support participation from all group members

[23]. Without that inclusion, diversity alone is not enough… and may even hinder creative problem solving.

Time, too, speaks loudly in healthcare. If time for creative exploration is always postponed, truncated, or treated as low priority, people get the message that ideation is optional or frivolous. When institutions protect time for reflection, whether in safety huddles, workshops, or post-event reviews, and then act on those ideas, it sends a powerful signal that creative thinking is part of how care improves, not a distraction from it.

Creating conditions for creativity in healthcare teams is therefore not a matter of trying to make clinical work resemble a design studio. It is a matter of recognizing what forms of environment, participation, and facilitation allow different kinds of knowledge to enter the room. In patient safety, that distinction has practical consequences because the quality of ideas generated depends heavily on who feels able to contribute, under what conditions, and at what point in the process.

## Applying Creative Tools in Patient Safety

The principles and conditions outlined above gain clarity when observed in practice. Ideation methods often appear abstract until grounded in the operational realities of care delivery. The following illustrative examples demonstrate how structured creativity can reshape familiar safety challenges. These scenarios are hypothetical but reflect common dynamics in clinical environments.

Each example illustrates a different movement: inversion to expose vulnerability, perspective-shifting to integrate stakeholder experience, and structured modification to redesign entrenched workflows. The intent is not to present idealized solutions but to show how disciplined ideation can transform stalled conversations into actionable direction.

## Example 1: Reverse Brainstorming to Address Missed Abnormal Labs

A large internal medicine team had identified a recurring issue during safety reviews: abnormal lab results, particularly critical potassium levels and pending cultures, were sometimes missed when patients were transferred from inpatient to skilled nursing facilities. Despite implementing standard discharge summaries and checklists, lapses continued to occur.

The safety team decided to try a reverse brainstorming session. Instead of asking, "How can we ensure critical labs are followed up after discharge?" the facilitator posed the prompt: "How could we guarantee that abnormal labs are missed during transitions?"

Participants responded with ideas like:

- Don't include pending labs in the discharge summary.
- Assume the receiving facility will check the labs.
- Send discharge paperwork after the patient has already left.
- Avoid assigning responsibility for lab follow-up.

When the group reflected on their responses, several uncomfortable truths emerged. Many of these "worst-case" ideas resembled real behaviors, like relying on faxed documentation, assuming responsibility would transfer implicitly, and failing to flag critical values in the electronic health record (EHR).

This exercise prompted a redesign of the discharge planning process. The team added a visual flag for pending critical results, assigned explicit follow-up ownership before discharge, and embedded a "pending results handoff" section into the EHR template. Within three months, missed critical result incidents during transitions had decreased significantly. Just as importantly, the team developed a new appreciation for the friction points in handoffs—and a practical way to surface and solve them.

## Example 2: Role-Storming with Personas to Improve Alarm Responses

On a telemetry unit in a community hospital, clinicians were struggling with alarm fatigue. Alarms were being ignored, silenced, or missed, and a recent patient safety review revealed several near misses. The team held an ideation session using role-storming, leveraging several previously developed personas (based on real consumer insight and employee data). Instead of ideating as themselves, participants role-played as "Marcus," a seasoned night nurse juggling six patients with varying acuity, and "Tanya," a family caregiver unfamiliar with medical technology.

From Marcus' perspective, ideas emerged around customizable alarm escalation paths and visual dashboards that surfaced the most urgent alerts first, leveraging patient-specific analytics. From Tanya's perspective, suggestions included a caregiver-facing screen showing which alarms had been acknowledged and by whom, reducing confusion and fear.

Role-storming helped the team imagine needs and solutions they might not have considered otherwise. It also illuminated how current processes privileged staff efficiency over patient and family experience. The session led to a joint initiative between nursing and the Information Services team to develop a prototype for alarm triage supported by visual cues.

## Example 3: SCAMPER to Rethink Patient Safety Communication Tools

A quality team wanted to revamp the tool used to document and communicate near misses but struggled to move beyond small format tweaks. During a retreat, they used the SCAMPER method, applying its structured lens to the current tool:

- *Substitute*: Could we replace written reporting with voice notes or visual storytelling?
- *Combine*: Could we combine safety reporting with team huddles or existing rounding forms?
- *Adapt*: Are there tools from aviation or nuclear safety that we could adapt?
- *Modify*: Could we modify the language to reflect more psychological safety and less blame?
- *Put to another use*: Could this data also inform onboarding or training?
- *Eliminate*: What if we removed the requirement to label severity up front?
- *Rearrange*: What if staff submitted stories first, and analysis happened later?

The process pushed the team beyond surface-level changes and into the realm of strategic reimagining. One prototype that emerged was a mobile app that allowed for anonymous, audio-based reporting, with prompts adapted from storyboarding tools. While still in development, the app has already spurred dialogue about transparency and frontline empowerment.

Each of these examples demonstrates how creative tools can move teams from analysis paralysis to meaningful momentum. The problems discussed are not new. But the methods used to engage with them are. When reframing and ideation are embedded in patient safety culture, even long-standing issues can become entry points for new insight and action.

## Conclusion

The quality of patient safety interventions depends in part on what happens between recognizing a problem and choosing a response. When that interval is compressed, teams often arrive quickly at options that are familiar, administratively legible, and easy to justify. Those options may still be weak. They may fit the organization more comfortably than they fit the problem.

Structured ideation changes that dynamic by keeping the field open long enough for a wider range of responses to emerge. It does not remove the need for judgment, feasibility, or constraint. It delays their dominance just enough to allow possibilities to be considered that might otherwise disappear before they are fully formed. In healthcare, where authority gradients and operational urgency shape how groups think together, that delay can matter a great deal.

These methods are useful not because they make safety work more creative in some general sense, but because they help teams avoid narrowing too soon around the most available solution. They create conditions in which the problem can exert more influence on the intervention than institutional habit does.

Ideas generated in this way remain provisional. They may be promising, but they have not yet encountered the conditions that will determine whether they can hold up in practice.

## References


1. Acar OA, Tuncdogan A, van Knippenberg D, Lakhani KR. Collective creativity and innovation: an interdisciplinary review, integration, and research agenda. Acad Manage Rev. 2024;49(1):42–71.
2. Capuano C, et al. A systematic review of research on conformity. Int Rev Soc Psychol. 2024;37(1):Article 874.
3. Ez-Zaouia M, Carrillo R. The group folding effect: the role of collaborative process structuring and social interaction in group work. ACM Trans Comput Hum Interact. 2023;30(4):1–31.
4. Diehl M, Stroebe W. Productivity loss in brainstorming groups: toward the solution of a riddle. J Pers Soc Psychol. 1987;53(3):497–509.
5. Paulus PB, Nijstad BA. Group creativity: innovation through collaboration. Oxford: Oxford University Press; 2003.
6. Adanez A. Does quantity generate quality? Testing the fundamental principle of brainstorming. Span J Psychol. 2005;8(2):215–20.
7. Nijstad BA, Stroebe W. How the group affects the mind: a cognitive model of idea generation in groups. Pers Soc Psychol Rev. 2006;10(3):186–213.
8. Karau SJ, Williams KD. Social loafing: a meta-analytic review and theoretical integration. J Pers Soc Psychol. 1993;65(4):681–706.

9. Edmondson AC, Bransby DP. Psychological safety comes of age: observed themes in an established literature. Annu Rev Organ Psychol Organ Behav. 2023;10:55–78.
10. Dorst K. Frame innovation: create new thinking by design. Cambridge, MA: MIT Press; 2015.
11. Martin R. The design of business: why design thinking is the next competitive advantage. Boston: Harvard Business Press; 2009.
12. Litcanu M, Prostean O, Oros C, Mnerie AV. Brain-writing vs. brainstorming case study for power engineering education. Procedia Soc Behav Sci. 2015;191:387–90.
13. De Dreu CKW. When too little or too much hurts: evidence for a curvilinear relationship between task conflict and innovation in teams. J Manage. 2019;45(5):2135–64.
14. Nemeth CJ, Personnaz M, Personnaz B, Goncalo JA. The liberating role of conflict in group creativity: a study in two countries. Eur J Soc Psychol. 2004;34(4):365–74.
15. Harvey S, Kou CY. Collective engagement in creative tasks: the role of evaluation and dissent. Acad Manage J. 2013;56(4):1141–63.
16. Stokes PD. Creativity from constraints: the psychology of breakthrough. New York: Springer; 2006.
17. Mullen B, Johnson C, Salas E. Productivity loss in brainstorming groups: a meta-analytic integration. Basic Appl Soc Psychol. 1991;12(1):3–23.
18. Michanek J, Breiler A. The idea agent: the handbook on creative processes. London: Routledge; 2014.
19. De Bono E. Lateral thinking: creativity step by step. New York: Harper & Row; 1970.
20. Eberle B. SCAMPER on: games for imagination development. Waco: Prufrock Press; 1996.
21. Ito A, Sato K, Yumoto Y, Sasaki M, Ogata Y. A concept analysis of psychological safety: further understanding for application to health care. Nurs Open. 2021;9(1):467–89.
22. O'Donovan R, McAuliffe E. A systematic review of factors that enable psychological safety in healthcare teams. Int J Qual Health Care. 2020;32(4):240–50.
23. Vedres B, Vasarhelyi O. Inclusion unlocks the creative potential of gender diversity in teams. Sci Rep. 2023;13:29670.

# Prototyping for High Reliability

# 6

## Introduction

When the term *prototype* is used in healthcare, it often suggests a polished device, a digital product, or a near-finished intervention moving toward implementation. In patient safety work, the term is more practical and more provisional. A prototype is a way of testing assumptions before they harden into policy, workflow, or institutional expectation.

In this setting, prototyping is intentionally rough, rapid, and low-cost. Its purpose is not to perfect a tool or process in advance, but to make a proposed change tangible enough to examine. A prototype may take the form of a sketched handoff tool, a role-played discharge conversation, a mock-up of a room layout, or a brief simulation of a revised workflow. What matters is not polish. What matters is whether the intervention can be made concrete enough to reveal where it creates confusion, where it adds burden, how people respond to it, and what still needs to change.

Design literature often distinguishes between low-fidelity and high-fidelity prototypes. Low-fidelity, or "lo-fi," prototypes are quick, inexpensive, and intentionally incomplete. They are used to invite critique, surface hidden assumptions, and identify weaknesses before significant resources are committed. High-fidelity, or "hi-fi," prototypes more closely resemble the intended final form. They may include realistic materials, fuller workflows, or


K. Rasmussen, *Rethinking Patient Safety*,
https://doi.org/10.1007/978-3-032-26054-3_6

more developed digital interfaces. In patient safety work, inquiry often begins with low-fidelity methods because they allow teams to learn quickly while limiting unnecessary exposure for patients and staff [1].

This orientation aligns closely with high-reliability science. Reliability does not require eliminating every small failure in advance. It depends on building systems that can anticipate, contain, and learn from failure without allowing that failure to become consequential harm [2]. Prototyping serves that purpose by treating proposed changes as hypotheses about system behavior rather than as finished solutions awaiting rollout. Testing those hypotheses under controlled conditions allows organizations to learn before they commit themselves to full operational exposure.

Prototyping also supports organizational learning at a deeper level. It does more than refine a single intervention. It draws attention to the assumptions embedded in design decisions, to the conditions under which work is actually performed, and to the system features that make safe performance easier or harder to sustain. In that sense, prototyping is both a practical step in implementation and a way of examining how safety is being produced in practice.

Its value in patient safety lies partly in the change from abstraction to encounter. Instead of debating possible solutions at a distance, teams interact with provisional versions of them, observe what happens, and gather feedback from frontline staff, patients, and caregivers. The result is not simply a better tool. It is a more informed understanding of the system into which that tool is being introduced.

Before turning to specific methods, it is useful to distinguish prototyping from other forms of change activity.

**Important**
A prototype asks, *What breaks, and why?* A pilot asks, *Does this perform reliably under real conditions?* Implementation asks, *Can this be sustained at scale?*

**Table 6.1** Key distinctions between prototypes, pilots, and implementation

| Term | Primary purpose | Risk exposure | Typical scope |
|---|---|---|---|
| Prototype | Learn and refine the design | Minimal and tightly controlled | Small, experimental |
| Pilot | Evaluate readiness for broader rollout | Moderate and monitored | Limited real-world deployment |
| Implementation | Standardize and sustain change | System-wide | Multisite or organization-wide |

**Definition** Prototyping is a structured, iterative method used to test and refine safety interventions through the creation of preliminary, low-risk representations of a proposed process, tool, or workflow. Within patient safety science, prototyping functions as a mechanism for anticipatory learning, enabling teams to examine how an intervention performs under realistic conditions prior to formal adoption (Table 6.1).

This distinction matters. When organizations conflate prototypes with pilots, they prematurely expose patients and staff to untested change. Prototyping, by contrast, preserves reversibility. It creates a learning buffer between idea generation and operational commitment.

## Developing Low-Cost, Rapid Prototypes for Safety Interventions

In patient safety work, promising ideas often stall in discussion or move into practice too quickly without safeguards. Both patterns increase risk. Prototyping offers a third path: create a quick, inexpensive representation of an idea, observe its behavior, and revise it before scaling.

Low-cost prototyping emphasizes simplicity. The purpose is not to finalize a design but to make it visible enough for people to react to it. In practice, this might mean sketching a version of what a new service might look like and asking patients for feedback, mocking up a new process flow to walk through, or role-playing a high-risk conversation. Because these prototypes are intentionally incomplete, they reduce the pressure of perfection and invite honest critique. Early prototypes are valuable precisely because they make learning feel permissible and change reversible [1].

For patient safety teams, this approach is pragmatic as well as principled. It reinforces high-reliability behaviors such as noticing weak signals, resisting oversimplification, and learning from small failures before they become large ones [2]. Instead of assuming a process will work because it sounds reasonable on paper, teams can watch it unfold under realistic constraints and adapt while the cost of revision remains low.

## Approaches to Lo-Fi Prototyping in Healthcare

### Sketching and Storyboarding`

One of the simplest and most effective ways to begin prototyping is to put pen to paper. A sketch or paper mock-up makes an abstract idea visible and concrete, which invites feedback in a way that words alone cannot. For example, drawing the layout of a new bedside handoff form quickly reveals whether the flow makes sense or whether critical fields are easy to find. Storyboarding builds on this approach by illustrating how a process unfolds step by step. A storyboard might use a series of small sketches or boxes to show how a patient moves through a discharge process or how a nurse and physician interact during a handoff. The purpose is not artistic quality but clarity. By walking through a storyboard, teams can identify where confusion, delays, or risks of error might arise.

Once sketches or storyboards exist, they can be shared with others for quick, structured feedback. For example, a facilitator might show staff a draft handoff form and ask, "What is the first thing you would do with this? Where do your eyes go first? What seems missing or unnecessary?" These questions encourage honest critique and generate insight that would not surface in a theoretical discussion.

Use cases for sketches and storyboarding in patient safety include:

- Drafting a new risk assessment form that new patients will complete on a mobile phone to ensure it is intuitive before adding it to a digital application
- Visualizing the sequence of steps in a central line insertion to identify where errors or omissions are most likely
- Sketching a patient discharge packet to see if patients and caregivers understand the order of information and can easily locate what they need
- Mapping the communication steps between pharmacy, patients and their caregivers, and nursing when reviewing medications during a home health visit.

These simple tools lower the barrier to participation. Staff who might not feel comfortable critiquing a policy document often feel more at ease marking up a sketch or suggesting how to rearrange a storyboard. In this way, sketches create a low-pressure environment that prioritizes learning over perfection.

## Cards and Wireframes for Digital Processes

Electronic health records (EHR) are a frequent focus of patient safety interventions, yet they are notoriously difficult to change. A common trap is to move directly into system build requests, which consume time and resources before the design has been validated. Low-fidelity prototyping provides a safer path.

One method is to represent each EHR step with index cards or sticky notes. Each card might stand for a documentation field, a decision point, or an order set. Staff can arrange and rearrange the cards on a table to mimic the sequence of actions they would take in the EHR. This "paper EHR" approach makes the invisible workflow visible. It allows teams to identify redundancies, missing fields, or confusing sequences long before anyone touches the actual system.

Wireframing takes this one step further. A wireframe is a simple, stripped-down sketch of a digital screen or page layout. Wireframes can be drawn on paper, created with basic software, or even mocked up on whiteboards. They omit details like color or final design, focusing instead on placement of elements and flow.

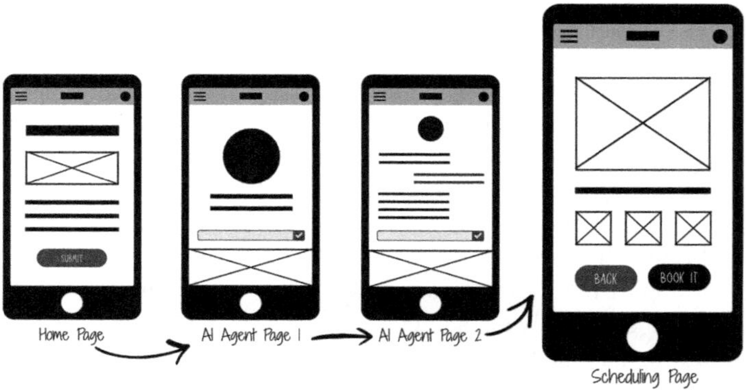


**Fig. 6.1** An example of a wireframe illustrating a patient health portal interface. The wireframe highlights layout, information hierarchy, and flow without visual design detail, allowing teams to explore an idea prior to a digital build or integration into the live system

For example, a wireframe of a medication reconciliation screen might show where drug names, dosing, and confirmation buttons appear, without worrying about fonts or colors (Fig. 6.1).

Both cards and wireframes are powerful because they allow for quick iteration. A facilitator can walk a clinician through the prototype, asking questions such as: "Where would you click next? What do you expect to happen here? What feels unnecessary?" Their answers often surface mismatches between designer intent and user expectation. Because the prototype is low-cost and non-technical, changes can be made in minutes rather than weeks.

Here are a few examples of use cases for cards and wireframes in patient safety:

- Redesigning a sepsis order set to ensure critical actions are visible and prioritized
- Testing the usability of a new documentation flow for bedside handoff on a mobile device before building it in the EHR
- Exploring ways to streamline medication reconciliation by mapping each required step on cards
- Visually prototyping an alert system for abnormal lab results to ensure it grabs attention without overwhelming staff

These techniques shift the conversation from abstract frustration ("the system doesn't work for us") to concrete redesign. They also democratize the process, giving frontline staff and patients the ability to shape EHR workflows without needing technical expertise.

### Scenario Role-Play

Many people think of role-play as a training exercise, but in prototyping, it becomes something more powerful. It allows teams to step into the perspective of others and test how safety interventions hold up under different conditions. When paired with personas, introduced in Chap. 3, role-play shifts from performance to exploration.

Personas provide a structured way to represent the diverse experiences of patients, families, and staff. In role-play, these personas come to life. A nurse might be asked to role-play "Marcus," a patient balancing multiple chronic conditions and medication regimens. A physician might play "Elena," a patient facing language barriers and relying on translated materials to understand instructions. Another staff member might step into the role of a caregiver who is anxious, exhausted, and skeptical. Acting out a new handoff process, a discharge conversation, or a rapid response activation with these personas exposes breakdowns that would never be obvious in a meeting.

Role-play with personas also uncovers assumptions. Staff often discover that they are using jargon that patients cannot understand, making eye contact only with colleagues and not with caregivers, or rushing through explanations that require more time. These observations can then be fed back into prototype refinement.

Facilitators can strengthen this process by asking targeted questions during or after the role-play, such as:

- "What assumptions were you making about what this patient or colleague understood?"
- "How did it feel to experience this process from the perspective of the persona?"
- "Where did tension, confusion, or frustration emerge?"

The following are examples of role-playing leveraging personas to strengthen patient safety efforts:

- Testing a hospital-at-home discharge process with personas representing patients whose primary language is not English.
- Rehearsing handoffs between physicians and medical assistants while assigning personas that highlight power dynamics or communication barriers.
- Exploring an informed consent workflow for interventional radiology by role-playing from the hospitalist, radiologist, nursing, and patient perspectives.
- Stress-testing a rapid response activation by assigning personas that represent an inexperienced nurse, a delayed physician, or a distressed family member.

By connecting role-play to personas, organizations move beyond simply "acting it out." The exercise becomes a structured method for stress-testing processes through the lens of diverse patient and staff experiences. This approach challenges hidden assumptions, exposes blind spots, and surfaces risks that are often invisible in traditional reviews. It also deepens empathy, helping teams appreciate the emotional, cognitive, and practical realities of those living the process. Most importantly, role-play with personas generates actionable insights that can be fed directly into prototype refinement, ensuring that interventions are technically sound and also human-centered and safer in practice.

### Environmental Walk-Throughs

The physical environment plays a critical role in patient safety, yet changes to space are often made without testing how people will actually move, see, or reach within it. Environmental prototyping applies staged experimentation to space: start rough, learn quickly, and increase fidelity only when evidence warrants it. The aim is to surface hazards, friction, and flow constraints before capital is committed. Use structured safety tools to guide what you look for and how you decide next steps, for example, the Agency for Healthcare Research and Quality's (AHRQ) Safety Risk Assessment domains and methods from Failure Mode and

Effect Analysis [3, 4]. Evidence from healthcare design research and simulation can then be used to pressure test alternatives as fidelity increases [5–7].

To put this into practice, begin with fast, low-cost trials and progress to higher fidelity only when learning justifies it. The approaches below are ordered from lighter to heavier footprints. Select the lightest method that answers your question, then combine or escalate as needed.

- *Low-fidelity, move-fast set-ups.* Use painter's tape, cardboard, rolling carts, and temporary signage to block out proposed layouts. Walk through typical tasks in the mocked space while a facilitator times steps, counts interruptions, and documents reach distances and line of sight. Inject likely failure points on purpose, for example, a missing supply or a partially blocked monitor, to observe how the team detects and recovers [4].
- *Pop-up micro-units.* Convert an unused room or corner into a pop-up lab for 24–72 h. Stock it with real or simulated equipment, then run scheduled scenarios, including surge moments like shift change. Debrief each run, change one variable at a time, and rerun. This creates rapid learning cycles without capital expense.
- *Wayfinding and visibility trials.* Prototype wayfinding by placing temporary signs and floor markers. Invite staff, patients, or volunteers to navigate common routes, for example, parking to registration to infusion, while observers capture detours and delays. Test lines of sight from nurses' stations using placeholders for monitors and curtains. Use the AHRQ Safety Risk Assessment lens to check systematically for infection control, falls hazards, behavioral health safety, medication safety, security, and patient handling issues [3].
- *3P full-scale mock-ups.* For decisions with significant impact, run a production preparation process (3P) session. Build full-scale room or clinic mock-ups with cardboard and foam, script work choreography in the space, and iterate layouts across multiple cycles in a single day. 3P brings frontline staff and patients into the room to co-design flow, adjacencies, and placement before any build is authorized [5].

- *Simulation for space and process.* Use clinical simulation to evaluate how a space supports teamwork and safety. Run realistic cases through the mocked environment, pause to debrief, and log latent safety threats and usability issues. Pair space trials with targeted checks for any new tools or handoffs you are testing [6].
- *End-to-end journey walk-throughs.* Prototype the experience from threshold to threshold, not only inside a room. Walk through a complete journey for a realistic persona, for example, from arrival at imaging to the inpatient unit to discharge. Carry what they would carry, stop where they would stop, and read what they would read. Storyboard the sticking points, then return to the pop-up space to address them.

Another approach to consider is overlaying Failure Mode and Effect Analysis to any of the trials above to make risks explicit and decisions actionable [4, 8]. Keep it fast, visual, and sized to the sandbox pace. Start by mapping the scenario in five to seven steps, then list potential failure modes and effects for each step, along with likely causes and current controls. Use the FMEA severity and probability matrix to assign a hazard score, and the decision tree to determine whether action is needed given detectability, existing controls, and potential for harm. Design controls that eliminate, substitute, engineer, simplify, standardize, or add checks, with preference for physical and visual controls when the environment is the driver. Build each control into the mock-up, rerun the scenario, and note residual risk and observed effects. Decide in advance what signals matter, for example, reach distances, line of sight confirmation, task time, interruptions, handoffs, and opportunities for error, then capture both quantitative counts and qualitative quotes. Feed findings into the next iteration the same day. When a configuration performs well in the pop-up and in simulation, graduate to a tightly scoped sandbox trial on one shift before any pilot or capital spend.

Taken together, these practices turn space decisions into learning cycles. The combination of low-cost mock-ups, structured safety checks, targeted simulation, and computer-based flow modeling reduces risk while increasing adoption. Staff see their input reflected in the design. Leaders see evidence, not opinion, before they commit resources.

## Simulation Exercises

Most healthcare teams are familiar with the use of simulation for education and competency assessment. In prototyping, simulation serves a different purpose. It becomes a safe experiment that pressures a draft design so you can see where it fails, why it fails, and how to fix it before anyone depends on it in practice. The primary question is not "did people perform correctly," it is "does this new tool or workflow hold up under realistic conditions, and what must change next" [6, 9].

When it comes to patient safety and high reliability, the approach is different. Simulation prototypes must be designed to answer a hypothesis, not to certify skills. State the learning target in one line, for example, "Will the revised sepsis order set reduce time to antibiotics by 5 min during peak volume?" Stage the real conditions that make work hard, for example, interruptions, partial information, language barriers, alarms, and competing priorities. Design the scenario so you can see the system, for example, time to key steps, omissions in handoff, number of clarifying questions, etc. Prebrief the team that the prototype is under test, then debrief to redesign the prototype, not to grade the people. Make at least one change and run a second cycle the same day. This turns simulation into an iterative design engine, not a one-time event [6].

High-reliability science emphasizes preoccupation with failure, sensitivity to operations, and learning before harm occurs. Simulation-as-prototype operationalizes these principles. You invite failure in a controlled space, pay attention to how work really happens, and convert breakdowns into design changes that strengthen the system. Debriefing becomes a mechanism for organizational learning rather than personal critique. The signal you seek is improved reliability of the process, not individual heroics [2].

Many organizations run a single high-fidelity drill, collect generic feedback, then move on. Instead, script two or three fast cycles that each answer one design question. Capture only the measures you will act on today. Build debrief notes directly into change decisions, for example, revise the handoff script wording, move a supply, change a button location in the mock EHR, and adjust roles for clarity. Treat interruptions and variability as deliberate test variables, not as noise to be eliminated. Pair in-situ runs with the environmental mock-ups discussed earlier, so you see how space, tools, and people interact. When the concept performs reliably in simulation, move it to a controlled sandbox on one unit or shift before any pilot [3, 9].

### Rapid Field Trials

A rapid field trial is a short, bounded experiment in live care that answers one question and reduces uncertainty before anyone depends on a new design. It is not a pilot. A pilot seeks confirmation about the spread. A rapid field trial seeks truth about what breaks, what holds, and what must change next [10, 11].

When it comes to rapid field testing, it's important to keep the design simple and protective. Keep the boundary for testing cycles narrow: one unit, one shift, or a fixed number of cases. Put clear protections in place: criteria, visible stop rules, a named point person at the bedside if anything is unclear, etc. Identify what measures will be collected. Focus on only the measures you can act on immediately (the same day), for example, time to a critical step, omissions in required content, interruptions, visible workarounds, etc.

Run the trial as a short sequence that repeats quickly:

1. State the hypothesis and the success signal.
2. Prebrief that the process is on trial, not the people.
3. Run the work under realistic conditions, including interruptions and competing priorities.
4. Debrief to change the design, not to grade performance.
5. Rerun the trial the same day to test the change you just made.

This cadence embodies high-reliability principles. It invites failure in a controlled way, keeps attention on how work actually happens, and converts breakdowns into design changes before harm can occur.

The following brief example illustrates the cadence. An emergency department wants to know whether a revised sepsis pathway will shorten the time to first antibiotic during peak volumes. The boundary is one pod for six consecutive cases. Stop rules and a reversion plan are posted in the nurses' station. Observers time triage to order, order to pharmacy verification, and verification to administration. They track clarifying questions, task stacking, and missed criteria. After two cases are completed, the team moves a key prompt earlier in triage and relocates a supply that caused a delay. A second cycle confirms the change. A third cycle adds a planned interruption to see whether the pathway still holds. Only after the design performs reliably across cycles does the team consider a larger test.

Most organizations skip rapid field trials and move straight to a pilot. Replace that habit with two or three rapid cycles. Pair each cycle with the prototypes you created earlier so people, process, and space are tested together. When the concept holds under varied conditions, extend the window or the volume. Only then, prepare a true pilot with defined success and balanced measures. This is how small tests become reliable designs without gambling on a full go-live.

## Hi-Fi Prototyping for Patient Safety

Some questions cannot be answered with sketches, index cards, or tabletop walk-throughs. High-fidelity prototyping increases realism so teams can see how a design holds under pressure, across roles, and within the digital and physical systems that shape care. Where low-fidelity work asks, "Does this idea make sense?" high-fidelity prototyping asks, "What actually happens when real people interact with this under realistic conditions?" The goal remains learning, not polish. Teams should move to higher fidelity when the next critical question depends on realistic cues, integrated workflows, or near-live coordination, and step back down when a simpler method will suffice.

High-fidelity prototyping emphasizes completeness and context. It tests whether a design functions when time is constrained, interruptions occur, documentation requires specific EHR sequences, and equipment or layout influences performance. In patient safety, these contextual variables are not peripheral. They are often where risk emerges. Safety failures rarely result from flawed intentions alone. They arise from the interaction between design and operational complexity, a dynamic well-documented in systems-based safety science [12–14].

For that reason, high-fidelity testing should be anchored in a clearly defined hypothesis. Rather than asking generally whether a solution "works," teams specify what reliability question is being tested. For example:

- Will the revised handoff protocol reduce omissions in critical patient information during peak census?
- Does the redesigned discharge workflow improve patient comprehension without increasing task time?
- Will the new order set reduce time to antibiotic administration without increasing alert overrides?

High-fidelity prototyping is therefore not an exercise in confirmation. It is a disciplined method for testing whether a design maintains safety under realistic stress.

Reliable systems anticipate failure, remain sensitive to operations, and learn before harm occurs [2, 15]. High-fidelity tests operationalize these principles by deliberately introducing realistic conditions and observing how the design responds. Friction points, work-arounds, delays, and unintended consequences surface while the intervention remains provisional and reversible [16, 17].

### Test-Environment EHR Builds and User Acceptance Testing

When a proposed safety intervention involves digital workflow changes, teams should build the new order set, documentation flow, or alert in a non-production EHR environment. This allows for user acceptance testing (UAT) before live exposure.

UAT is a structured evaluation in which representative clinicians, pharmacists, and staff use the tool under realistic conditions to determine whether it supports safe, efficient work. It differs from vendor testing or technical quality assurance. Those processes verify that the system functions. UAT evaluates whether the system functions for clinicians during real operations.

Each UAT cycle should begin with a defined hypothesis and a success signal. For example:

- Will this build reduce omissions in required documentation fields?
- Does the revised screen layout decrease navigation backtracking?
- Will the alert timing reduce unnecessary overrides during peak workload?

Clear hypotheses prevent UAT from devolving into general usability feedback and, instead, tie testing directly to safety performance.

Testing scenarios should reflect actual workflow conditions. Sample charts should include realistic medications, allergies, active problems, lab values, pending tasks, and handoffs such as pharmacy verification or discharge instructions. Users should walk the entire workflow from start to finish rather than test isolated screens.

During UAT, teams may use the 2025 SAFER Guides as a structured lens to examine safety vulnerabilities related to data entry, decision support, communication, contingency planning, and system resilience [18]. This ensures that usability feedback is evaluated alongside known EHR safety risk domains.

### UAT Observation

Observation during UAT focuses on how clinicians navigate the system under realistic cognitive and operational load. The goal is to identify where the design strengthens reliability and where it introduces risk.

Observers should document behaviors tied to time, screen, and task sequence. Brief clarifying questions may be asked to understand why a specific action occurred. The following are things to watch for:

- *First-glance behavior on each screen*: where eyes go first and what users try to do next
- *Navigation path*: extra clicks, backtracks, dead ends, and duplicate entries
- *Hesitation points*: where users pause, reread, or ask for help, and why
- *Required content*: omissions, when they occur, and what made completion of the task challenging
- *Prompts and alerts*: clarity, timing, relevance, overrides, and alert pileups
- *Field order and defaults*: whether the order of fields matches the real workflow and whether defaulted content helps or misleads
- *Information handoffs*: how data moves to and from pharmacy, lab, imaging, and discharge instructions, and where it breaks
- *Consistency across roles and devices*: whether the same task works for nurses, physicians, and pharmacists on desktop and mobile
- *Recovery after interruption*: how quickly users find their place and what is lost
- *Time to key steps and variation*: averages and spread across cases
- *Patient-facing content*: accuracy and readability of printouts and instructions
- *Accessibility and language support*: font size, contrast, and interpreter workflows for patients whose primary language is not English
- *Work-arounds*: improvised steps users invent to finish the task, and what those reveal

**Important**
The guiding question throughout UAT remains consistent: Does this design reduce risk under realistic use, or does it create new points of fragility?

Use the SAFER Guides as a short checklist during any UAT observation so safety issues related to data entry, decision support, and communication are visible while you test [18].

## Digital Flow Modeling

Digital flow modeling allows teams to test operational hypotheses before changing physical space or staffing patterns. A simplified spreadsheet model may estimate queues and wait times, while discrete-event simulation tools capture variability and resource interactions [6, 7]. Models should be seeded with real operational data, including arrival rates, task time distributions, staffing levels, room capacity, and process constraints (an example is holding one bed open as part of a process). Many organizations already have these inputs in operational dashboards, data warehouses, or digital twins, which can provide realistic distributions and scenarios.

Each modeling effort should begin with a focused operational hypothesis. For example:

- Will this revised triage configuration reduce average time to first provider contact without increasing downstream congestion?
- Does holding one bed open for rapid admission reduce boarding time variability?
- Will consolidating discharge documentation reduce afternoon bottlenecks?

The model outputs predicted wait times, utilization rates, queue lengths, and blocking points. These results guide which configurations should move to physical mock-up or sandbox testing. Modeling does not replace live testing; it narrows options and reduces unnecessary risk before physical experimentation.

### AI-Generated Interactive Personas

Large language models can serve as simulated patients or caregivers for conversational prototyping. These tools allow teams to test communication design hypotheses before interacting with real patients. Use the persona foundations from Chap. 3, then bring them to life in a short, guided conversation.

Each AI-based prototype should begin with a clearly defined testing question. Based on that question, develop fictional personas and scenarios that will pressure test the experience. Include goals, concerns, health literacy, primary language, and emotional context. Give the model clear boundaries, for example, "respond only as the patient or caregiver, do not give medical advice," and specify the task, such as bedside handoff, discharge teach-back, or a scheduling call regarding an outpatient procedure. Participants conduct the interaction as they would during clinical care. Observations focus on comprehension gaps, pacing, language clarity, teach-back duration, and breakdown points. The script is revised immediately and retested.

Possible use cases for AI-generated personas in patient safety include:

- Practicing discharge instructions with a persona whose primary language is not English, including interpreter steps and translated materials
- Rehearsing an informed consent discussion with a worried caregiver who asks for plain-language explanations and risks in context
- Stress-testing a revised handoff script with a persona who interrupts, asks for clarification, or misremembers medications

Important safeguards: never include protected health information or real patient identifiers in prompts. Use only tools that your organization has approved, and follow organizational policies on data handling, logging, and retention. Treat model outputs as test inputs, not as clinical guidance, and watch for bias by rotating personas across language, literacy, disability, and cultural contexts. Align this practice with recognized governance frameworks and organizational AI policy, including risk management and validation expectations [19–21].

These conversational trials are fast and inexpensive, and they expose clarity and evaluate communication reliability. They do not replace UAT in a test EHR or simulation in space. Use them to refine wording, sequence, and comprehension, then graduate successful scripts to higher-fidelity tests where safety, integration, and handoffs are validated end to end.

## 3D Modeling and Virtual Reality Environments

Three-dimensional models and virtual reality (VR) let teams experience a proposed design at full scale before it exists. The purpose is not visual polish; it's to learn how people move, see, decide, and coordinate under realistic conditions, then change the design while changes are still inexpensive. Use these tools when patient safety is dependent on the line of sight, reach, congestion, movement choreography, or cross-role coordination.

Use cases for 3D and VR in patient safety include:

- Testing room layouts for visibility, reach, and equipment placement during emergencies
- Evaluating triage and treatment bay configurations for congestion and line of sight
- Rehearsing end-to-end workflows that cross departments so handoffs and waits are visible
- Prototyping wayfinding systems and signage to reduce navigational errors and travel time
- Preparing operational dress rehearsals that include pharmacy, transport, imaging, environmental services, and admitting so the choreography is realistic [5]

3D and VR prototypes focus on people in space. They answer questions about movement, visibility, access, and coordination. An EHR test build answers questions about data, logic, and handoffs between systems. These two approaches to prototyping are complementary. Teams may use VR or 3D modeling to settle layout and flow, then move to user acceptance testing in a non-production EHR to validate orders, documentation, and alerts before any live exposure.

3D modeling and VR are far more accessible than a decade ago, yet they still require time, skilled facilitation, and basic technical setup. Headset hygiene, motion sensitivity, and safe use policies need attention. Integration with building models and scheduling systems can be helpful but is not required for useful learning. Looking ahead, digital twins and real-time data streams are making it possible to couple virtual walk-throughs with live or simulated demand, which can narrow options before you build a physical mock-up. Remote co-design is also improving, which allows frontline staff from multiple sites to walk the same virtual unit together and make decisions in one session. Use your organization's approved software and follow local policies for procurement, data handling, and infection control for shared devices.

High-fidelity prototyping strengthens design integrity under realistic stress, but it does not yet answer the question of sustained performance in live care. Once a design demonstrates stability in simulation, UAT, digital modeling, or immersive environmental testing, the next question shifts from functionality to reliability: Will this hold when real variability enters the system? That transition requires a different learning structure.

## Sandboxes for Safety: Testing Solutions Before Implementation

High-fidelity prototyping increases realism, but it does not yet answer the question of how an intervention behaves in bounded live use. That is the function of the sandbox.

A sandbox is a structured, limited environment in which a more developed intervention can be tested under real conditions while exposure remains deliberately constrained. It occupies the space between prototype and pilot. In patient safety terms, it allows teams to examine whether the intervention remains stable when it encounters actual variability in staffing, interruptions, workload, and patient complexity.

This phase reflects core principles from high-reliability science. High-reliability organizations demonstrate preoccupation with failure, sensitivity to operations, and commitment to resilience [2]. A sandbox operationalizes these principles by inviting small-scale exposure specifically to surface weak signals prior to escalation. Successful simulation does not guarantee field reliability. The sandbox acknowledges that complexity increases once a design enters an authentic workflow.

The sandbox also aligns directly with the Model for Improvement, which emphasizes iterative testing through rapid Plan-Do-Study-Act cycles before broad implementation [10, 11]. The purpose is not confirmation but disciplined learning. Each sandbox cycle should be explicitly hypothesis-driven. For example:

- Does the redesigned handoff reduce omissions during night shift without increasing report duration?
- Does the revised sepsis pathway maintain time-to-antibiotics during peak census?
- Does the new discharge script improve teach-back accuracy without extending discharge time?

Framing the sandbox around measurable reliability questions prevents it from becoming an informal rollout. It remains a controlled experiment.

Many patient safety failures arise not from flawed intentions, but from untested assumptions about how work unfolds in context [14, 17]. Organizational learning theory emphasizes the importance of feedback loops that connect action to consequence in real time [22]. A sandbox creates those loops in compressed form. It transforms conceptual confidence into observed performance and allows redesign while revision costs remain low.

A well-constructed sandbox includes:

1. A clearly articulated reliability hypothesis
2. Explicit boundaries, such as one unit, one shift, or a fixed number of cases
3. Stop rules and reversion plans
4. Real-time monitoring tied to decision thresholds
5. Immediate review and redesign cycles

The point is not to confirm success. The point is to detect where the intervention still depends on hidden assumptions.

### Simulation Labs in Operational Context

Simulation can function as a sandbox when conducted in situ or in environments that closely reproduce real operational conditions. Rather than validating skills, these sessions test whether the intervention holds under real pressure. These can range from high-fidelity mannequin simulations to standardized patients or virtual environments. Simulation allows for the safe testing of interventions in situations that mimic the pressures, variability, and unpredictability of clinical care. Teams can rehearse handoffs, test new checklists, or experiment with communication tools under realistic conditions while still being able to pause, debrief, and redesign the system [2, 9].

### Tabletop Process Walk-Throughs with Live Parameters

Tabletop sandboxes extend beyond ideation into operational rehearsal. Multidisciplinary teams walk through real patient cases using the proposed workflow, identifying where mismatches between expectation and practice emerge. By slowing the process down and verbalizing each step, teams can uncover mismatched assumptions, bottlenecks, and potential failure points that would otherwise remain hidden.

### Parallel Testing

Parallel testing allows comparison between the current process and the proposed intervention within a small, controlled cohort.

This approach allows teams to measure differences directly. For example, a new medication reconciliation tool might be completed in tandem with the standard process for a small group of patients. Comparing results side by side in real time makes performance differences visible and reveals whether the prototype reduces errors, improves clarity, or creates new risks.

## Controlled Rollouts

A sandbox may take the form of a tightly bounded live trial in a single department or shift with continuous monitoring. Rather than spreading an intervention across multiple units, a sandbox rollout limits exposure. For example, a new bedside handoff script might be trialed during night shift only, with staff feedback collected daily. The tight boundary and active monitoring ensure that risks are contained while learning accumulates quickly.

Sandboxes provide more than technical data. They create psychological safety for staff who are asked to adopt change. When people see that an idea is being tested carefully and that their feedback matters, they are more likely to engage honestly. Sandboxes also provide leaders with tangible evidence of feasibility, risks, and potential benefits. They transform change from an abstract directive into a lived experience that can be observed, measured, and refined.

The Veterans Health Administration has demonstrated the value of this approach through its Diffusion of Excellence Initiative. The program identifies promising practices from across the Veterans Affairs (VA) system, then places them in structured testing environments where frontline teams adapt and evaluate them before broader rollout. By treating each site as a sandbox rather than jumping straight to systemwide adoption, the VA ensures that innovations are refined, risks are surfaced, and local context is respected [23]. This structured, iterative process illustrates how sandboxes can act as both a learning mechanism and a de-risking strategy in large healthcare organizations.

For patient safety, the lesson is clear: a sandbox is not a shortcut; it is a safeguard. It slows down the rush to implement by creating space to stress-test ideas and anticipate failure in advance. It builds staff confidence by signaling that change will not be imposed without rehearsal. And it equips leaders with the evidence needed to move forward responsibly. When organizations skip this step, they gamble with both safety and trust. When they commit to sandboxes, they create a pathway where solutions are tested, adapted, and proven reliable before they ever reach the bedside.

## Cross-Industry Prototyping Patterns That Transfer

The sequence outlined above (prototype, stress test, sandbox, then scale) is not unique to healthcare. It appears across other high-risk, high-variability sectors that must introduce change without magnifying unintended consequences. What transfers is not the specific artifact but the discipline of reversible experimentation.

Urban design, aviation, manufacturing, and digital infrastructure all provide examples of this logic. Changes are first introduced in temporary form, measured under actual conditions, revised in response to performance, and only then made permanent. These sequences mirror the learning patterns emphasized in high-reliability thinking: detect fragility early, expose systems to manageable stress, and learn before failure becomes catastrophic [1, 2].

The following case studies translate these patterns into patient safety language. Each example begins with problem recognition, moves through reversible testing, and culminates in scale only after measurable gains in safety and performance are demonstrated. The goal is not to import urban planning or software sprints into healthcare. It is to recognize the shared architecture of safe experimentation and apply it deliberately to clinical systems.

### Case Study 1: Paint Before Concrete—Broadway Redesign

When New York City confronted rising pedestrian injuries in Times and Herald Squares, the problem was not invisibility. The corridor was heavily trafficked, extensively engineered, and deeply studied. Yet observational data revealed persistent conflict between pedestrians and vehicles, diagonal intersections that increased crossing complexity, and sidewalks routinely overflowing into active travel lanes. NYC DOT documented that pedestrian injuries in the project area were significantly higher than in adjacent corridors, with crash patterns suggesting structural rather than behavioral causes [24, 25].

### Observe and Reframe

City planners reframed the problem from "How do we move more vehicles efficiently?" to "How do we make this corridor safer and more usable for the people already here?" This reframing was not rhetorical. It shifted the primary metric from car delay to injury reduction and pedestrian movement patterns. Public life studies documented pedestrian volumes reaching hundreds of thousands daily in Times Square, with measurable "pedlock" conditions during peak hours [24, 26]. The core insight was systems-based: the environment was misaligned with actual use.

### Create a Safe Sandbox

Rather than immediately committing to permanent reconstruction, the city closed sections of Broadway using reversible materials: paint, planters, movable barriers, and temporary seating. This allowed rapid reallocation of street space without structural demolition.

The intervention functioned as a live urban prototype. Traffic signal timing could be adjusted. Boundaries could be shifted. If results were unfavorable, the configuration could be reversed at minimal cost [25, 27]. The city effectively created a real-world sandbox.

### Measure What Matters

Evaluation was disciplined and public. Injury trends were tracked across all modes. In the project area, total injuries declined by 39% after implementation. Pedestrian injuries dropped by 40% in Times Square and 53% in Herald Square. Observers also recorded an 80% reduction in pedestrians walking in the roadway, a behavioral alignment signal [24].

Importantly, travel time analysis using taxi GPS data showed northbound travel improved by 17%, countering the assumption that safety gains would degrade efficiency [24, 25]. The prototype was judged by its operational performance, not its aesthetics.

### Iterate Before Exposure

Because materials were temporary, adjustments could be made rapidly. Planters shifted. Signage changed. Traffic flows were recalibrated. NACTO later codified this approach as interim design strategies, a practice that lets cities deliver near-term safety benefits while they continue to learn and refine the design before permanent construction [25]. Once the configuration produced consistent gains in safety and acceptable traffic performance, the city moved to higher-fidelity work and eventually permanent construction. The sequence was learn first, then build. That sequence maps directly to clinical governance, where measured improvements in safety and flow should precede any irreversible change.

### Why This Case Matters

The redesign illustrates disciplined prototyping at scale. The city observed real-world behavior, created reversible change, measured outcome signals tied to safety, iterated in public, and scaled only after reliability emerged. The work followed a recognizable arc: the city observed real-world behavior and reframed the problem, ideated inexpensive options, created a sandbox with clear boundaries, measured the signals that mattered, iterated quickly, and scaled only when performance was reliable. Each step de-risked the next. Stakeholders were part of the process, not just informed at the end. The measures were concrete, timely, and tied to decisions rather than collected for reports alone.

Healthcare teams can translate this playbook directly:

1. Start with observation in the real environment. Map where users naturally go and where conflicts occur. Reframe the question around ease and safety for the people in the flow today.
2. Use temporary, reversible materials to create a fast sandbox. Tape, carts, pop-up stations, and temporary signage change behavior tomorrow while keeping risk low.

3. Choose a short list of measures you can collect right away. In streets, those were injuries, speeds, volumes, and walking patterns. In care, use time to a critical step, completeness of required content, interruptions, recoveries from error, and teach-back success.
4. Iterate in public. Adjust the layout or script in days, not months, and show progress where the work happens.
5. Turn to permanence only when performance is both safer and stable under different conditions.

The Times and Herald Squares' work is not famous because it was bold. It is famous because it was careful. Paint came before concrete. That sequence is the essence of prototyping for patient safety, whether on a street or at the bedside.

## Case Study 2: Netflix's Chaos Engineering

Modern digital platforms operate in environments of extreme scale and interdependence. For Netflix, even minor system disruptions can affect millions of users simultaneously. Early reliability practices focused on redundancy and post-incident analysis. However, as infrastructure became more distributed and microservice-based, the organization recognized that hidden dependencies and cascading failures could remain undetected until a real outage occurred. Rather than waiting for spontaneous failure to reveal weaknesses, Netflix treated its production environment as a system that required proactive stress testing.

### Observe and Reframe

Netflix engineers reframed the problem from "How do we prevent outages?" to "How does our system behave when components fail?" This reflected a system's insight: in complex environments, failure is not an anomaly. Netflix serves hundreds of millions of users globally across a distributed cloud infrastructure. At that scale, failure is not rare; it is inevitable. The question is not whether components will break, but whether the system will continue to function safely and reliably when they do, and if the system can recover quickly.

### Create a Safe Sandbox

Rather than attempting to eliminate all failure in advance, Netflix adopted a different strategy: deliberately introducing controlled failures to understand how the system responds. This approach, known as Chaos Engineering, began with an internal tool called Chaos Monkey, which randomly terminated production instances to test whether services could recover without user disruption. The experiment was not reckless. It was bounded, monitored, and reversible. Its purpose was learning, not disruption [28, 29].

Failures were injected into the production environment during preselected windows and only after resilience safeguards were confirmed. The system was treated as a prototype under stress. This resembles healthcare simulation or sandbox testing, where the realism is preserved but the exposure is controlled.

### Measure What Matters

Each experiment was tied to explicit hypotheses. For example, if Service A failed, traffic should reroute within a specified latency threshold. Engineers tracked recovery time, customer-visible degradation, alert accuracy, cascading dependencies, and system load redistribution.

The emphasis was operational. Did the system behave as expected? Were signals detected quickly? Did safeguards activate reliably? When outcomes diverged from expectations, architectural vulnerabilities were revealed. These insights were documented, prioritized, and addressed before natural failures could expose them at scale [28, 29].

### Iterate Before Exposure

Chaos experiments were repeated after modifications to confirm resilience. Failure injection became routine practice rather than an exceptional testing. This institutionalized a learning cycle: stress, observe, adapt, retest. The sequence was deliberate: induce small, contained failures to prevent large, uncontrolled ones.

### Why This Case Matters

Netflix operationalized anticipatory learning. Instead of depending solely on post-incident reviews, the organization rehearsed disruption in advance. Structured stress testing revealed fragility, while consequences remained manageable.

Healthcare teams can translate this playbook directly:

1. Identify critical processes where failure would cascade.
2. Introduce controlled stress under monitored conditions.
3. Define measurable resilience indicators before testing.
4. Address vulnerabilities revealed during testing.
5. Repeat until performance stabilizes under variation.

The lesson is not about software. It is about discipline. Chaos was introduced deliberately so catastrophe would not occur accidentally. That sequence is the essence of high-fidelity prototyping in patient safety.

## Case Study 3: Clinical Systems Testing in a New Hospital

Opening a new hospital presents a unique safety paradox. Infrastructure may be complete, policies finalized, and staff trained. Yet the interaction between people, technology, workflow, and physical space remains untested under operational pressure. Latent safety threats can remain invisible until real patients enter the system.

In 2024, a multidisciplinary team applied Simulation-Based Clinical Systems Testing (SbCST) combined with Healthcare Failure Mode and Effect Analysis (HFMEA) to evaluate hospital readiness before admitting patients [30].

### Observe and Reframe

Rather than asking, "Is the hospital ready to open?" the team reframed the question to, "Where might this system fail under realistic clinical conditions?" This reframing shifted attention from compliance with construction checklists to operational performance under stress.

High-risk pathways were mapped, including emergency response activation, medication workflows, patient transport routes, interdepartmental communication, and escalation protocols. The building was treated as a provisional system rather than a finished product.

### Create a Safe Sandbox

Full-scale simulations were conducted in the actual clinical environment before opening. Interprofessional teams enacted realistic scenarios, including rapid deterioration events, communication escalations, handoffs, and equipment failures. Environmental stressors were introduced intentionally:

- Interruptions
- Competing task demands
- Time pressure
- Equipment access variability
- Role ambiguity

Observers focused on system performance rather than individual fault. The hospital functioned as a high-fidelity prototype.

### Measure What Matters

Observers documented latent safety threats, including equipment placement issues, unclear communication channels, workflow mismatches, and environmental barriers affecting response time. More than 75% of identified threats were mitigated prior to hospital opening [30]. Mitigations included:

- Relocating critical equipment
- Revising escalation pathways
- Clarifying documentation flow
- Adjusting team role assignments
- Modifying physical layout elements

Performance signals were tied directly to safety reliability rather than subjective readiness.

### Iterate Before Exposure

Simulations were repeated after modifications to confirm that vulnerabilities had been resolved. Testing cycles continued until the system demonstrated stable performance under variation. Patients entered a facility that had already been stressed safely.

### Why This Case Matters

This example demonstrates disciplined prototyping within healthcare itself. Entire facilities, workflows, and interdisciplinary interactions were treated as provisional until proven under operational stress.

Healthcare teams can translate this playbook directly:

1. Identify high-risk clinical pathways prior to implementation.
2. Conduct full-scale simulations in the real environment.
3. Define explicit performance and safety metrics before testing.
4. Document latent safety threats systematically.
5. Modify and retest until reliability stabilizes.

The work is methodical. Similar to the other case studies, the simulation preceded exposure, and learning preceded reliance. That sequence is the essence of prototyping in patient safety.

## Prototyping as Structured Anticipatory Learning

Taken together, these three cases show that prototyping is not a creative flourishing or a passing design trend. It is a disciplined method for managing risk in complex systems. Whether reallocating street space in Manhattan, injecting controlled failure into a global streaming platform, or stress-testing a hospital before opening its doors, the underlying logic remains strikingly consistent. Each system is treated as provisional. Interventions remain reversible, and judgment is tied to observable performance rather than conceptual appeal alone.

Across sectors, the sequence also holds. Organizations observe real behavior, reframe the problem around actual conditions of use, create a bounded testing environment, introduce structured stress, measure operational reliability, and scale only when performance begins to stabilize. The common thread is anticipatory learning. Failure is neither ignored nor treated only as something to punish after the fact. It is made visible in contained ways so that fragility can be identified while consequences remain manageable.

For patient safety, this changes the terms of improvement. The central question is not whether a proposed solution appears complete or administratively ready, but whether it has demonstrated reliability under realistic variation. That distinction matters. Policies may presume correctness. Prototypes test it.

When healthcare organizations prototype before implementation, they do more than refine tools or workflows. They acknowledge that design assumptions require testing, that stress can reveal what planning leaves hidden, and that small, contained breakdowns are preferable to large, uncontrolled harm. In that sense, prototyping is not peripheral to patient safety science. It is one of the more practical ways of acting on what the field has learned about complexity, fallibility, and system design.

The significance extends beyond any single intervention. Treating change as provisional until it has encountered the conditions of actual use introduces a different discipline into safety work, one that is less confident in abstraction and more willing to learn from exposure before commitment hardens. That posture becomes increasingly important once patient safety is considered not only as a matter of local redesign, but as a broader question of how organizations govern risk before harm forces recognition.

## References

1. Brown T. Change by design: how design thinking transforms organizations and inspires innovation. Boston: Harvard Business Press; 2009.
2. Weick KE, Sutcliffe KM. Managing the unexpected: sustained performance in a complex world. 3rd ed. San Francisco: Jossey-Bass; 2015.

3. Agency for Healthcare Research and Quality. Safety risk assessment toolkit for health care facility design. Rockville: AHRQ; 2026. Available from: https://www.ahrq.gov/patient-safety/settings/hospital/resource/safety-assess.html.
4. Institute for Healthcare Improvement. Patient safety essentials toolkit: failure modes and effects analysis (FMEA). Boston: IHI; 2017. Available from: https://www.ihi.org/sites/default/files/SafetyToolkit_FailureModesandEffectsAnalysis.pdf.
5. Ulrich RS, Zimring C, Zhu X, DuBose J, Seo H, Choi Y, et al. A review of the research literature on evidence-based healthcare design. HERD. 2008;1(3):61–125.
6. Agency for Healthcare Research and Quality. Simulation tool: workflow assessment for health IT toolkit. Rockville: AHRQ; 2026. Available from: https://digital.ahrq.gov/health-it-tools-and-resources/evaluation-resources/workflow-assessment-health-it-toolkit/all-workflow-tools/simulation.
7. Jun JB, Jacobson SH, Swisher JR. Application of discrete-event simulation in health care clinics: a survey. J Oper Res Soc. 1999;50:109–23.
8. VHA National Center for Patient Safety. Healthcare failure mode and effect analysis (HFMEA): step-by-step guidebook. Washington, DC: U.S. Department of Veterans Affairs; 2021. Available from: https://www.patientsafety.va.gov/docs/joe/Step-by-Step-Guidebook-HFMEA-January2021.pdf.
9. INACSL Standards Committee. The cornerstone healthcare simulation standards of best practice. Clin Simul Nurs. 2025;105:101774.
10. Institute for Healthcare Improvement. Model for improvement. Boston: IHI; 2026. Available from: https://www.ihi.org/library/model-for-improvement.
11. Langley GJ, Moen RD, Nolan KM, Nolan TW, Norman CL, Provost LP. The improvement guide: a practical approach to enhancing organizational performance. 2nd ed. San Francisco: Jossey-Bass; 2009.
12. Carayon P, Wetterneck TB, Rivera-Rodriguez AJ, Hundt AS, Hoonakker P, Holden R, et al. Human factors systems approach to healthcare quality and patient safety. Appl Ergon. 2014;45(1):14–25.
13. Reason J. Human error: models and management. BMJ. 2000;320(7237):768–70.
14. Lipsitz LA. Understanding health care as a complex system: the foundation for unintended consequences. JAMA. 2012;308(3):243–4.
15. Braithwaite J, Wears RL, Hollnagel E. Resilient health care: turning patient safety on its head. Int J Qual Health Care. 2015;27(5):418–20.
16. Ash JS, Sittig DF, Dykstra R, Campbell EM, Guappone KP, Dykstra RH. Some unintended consequences of clinical decision support systems. AMIA Annu Symp Proc. 2007;2007:26–30.
17. Cook RI, Render M, Woods DD. Gaps in the continuity of care and progress on patient safety. BMJ. 2000;320(7237):791–4.

18. Office of the National Coordinator for Health Information Technology. Safety assurance factors for EHR resilience (SAFER) guides. 2025 ed. Washington, DC: ONC; 2025. Available from: https://www.healthit.gov/topic/safety/safer-guides.
19. The Joint Commission, Coalition for Health AI. The responsible use of AI in healthcare (RUAIH). Oakbrook Terrace: The Joint Commission; 2025. Available from: https://www.jointcommission.org/en-us/knowledge-library/news/2025-09-jc-and-chai-release-initial-guidance-to-support-responsible-ai-adoption.
20. U.S. Food and Drug Administration, Health Canada, Medicines and Healthcare Products Regulatory Agency. Good machine learning practice for medical device development: guiding principles. Silver Spring: FDA; 2021. Available from: https://www.fda.gov/medical-devices/software-medical-device-samd/good-machine-learning-practice-medical-device-development-guiding-principles.
21. World Health Organization. Ethics and governance of artificial intelligence for health: guidance on large multi-modal models. Geneva: WHO; 2024.
22. Argyris C, Schön DA. Organizational learning II: theory, method, and practice. Reading: Addison-Wesley; 1995.
23. U.S. Department of Veterans Affairs, Veterans Health Administration. Diffusion of excellence playbook. Washington, DC: VHA; 2022.
24. New York City Department of Transportation. Green light for midtown: evaluation report. New York: NYC DOT; 2010. Available from: https://www.nyc.gov/html/dot/downloads/pdf/broadway_report_final2010_web.pdf.
25. National Association of City Transportation Officials. Urban street design guide: interim design strategies. New York: NACTO; 2025.
26. New York City Department of Transportation. World class streets: remaking New York City's public realm (Gehl Architects). New York: NYC DOT; 2008. Available from: https://www.nyc.gov/html/dot/downloads/pdf/WCS_Gehl_08_print.pdf.
27. Project for Public Spaces. Times Square project page. New York: PPS; 2026. Available from: https://www.pps.org/projects/times-square.
28. Basiri A, Behnam N, de Rooij R, Hochstein L, Kosewski L, Reynolds J, Rosenthal C. Chaos engineering. IEEE Softw. 2016;33(3):35–41.
29. Rosenthal C, Jones N, Basiri A. Chaos engineering: system resilience in practice. Sebastopol: O'Reilly Media; 2020.
30. Hazwani T, Hamam H, Caswell A, Madkhaly A, Al Saif S, Al Hassan Z, et al. Proactive patient safety: enhancing hospital readiness through simulation-based clinical systems testing and healthcare failure mode and effect analysis. Adv Simul. 2024;9(1):26. https://doi.org/10.1186/s41077-024-00298-z.

# 7 Beyond Cause Analysis: Proactive Patient Safety Frameworks

## Introduction

The modern patient safety movement has been learned by looking backward. Adverse events occur, organizations investigate them, and improvement efforts are built around what those investigations reveal. Root cause analysis (RCA), morbidity and mortality review, sentinel event investigation, and incident reporting have all contributed to that work. They have clarified important patterns of breakdown, drawn attention to latent conditions, and helped move the field away from simplistic accounts of individual blame.

Even when conducted rigorously, root cause analysis remains constrained by hindsight bias and by the tendency to translate nonlinear events into more manageable linear causal narratives [1]. Investigations often conclude with recommendations centered on additional training, policy reinforcement, or reminders. Those responses may be appropriate in some circumstances, but they rarely address deeper system design misalignments. As earlier discussion has suggested, harm often reflects accumulated latent conditions rather than a single visible failure point.

This limitation has become more difficult to ignore in complex clinical systems. A 2025 mixed-methods study comparing Safety-I and Safety-II approaches in primary care medication safety found that adverse-event-centered review captured only a portion of



K. Rasmussen, *Rethinking Patient Safety*,
https://doi.org/10.1007/978-3-032-26054-3_7

what shaped safety performance in practice [2]. When researchers examined work-as-done, they identified adaptive activities, compensatory routines, and system conditions that did not appear in retrospective event analysis alone. These findings are consistent with a broader shift in safety science: healthcare organizations cannot rely exclusively on visible failure as their primary teacher.

National patient safety frameworks have increasingly reflected the same concern. The Comprehensive Unit-based Safety Program, for example, emphasizes that systems are configured in ways that reliably produce the outcomes they generate [3]. When those outcomes are undesirable, corrective action aimed only at individual behavior or a single observed breakdown will often be insufficient. The system itself must become an object of examination.

A more proactive approach to patient safety begins with that recognition. It asks what happened after a breakdown and where vulnerability is already gathering in ordinary work. It broadens the object of inquiry from visible harm to the conditions that make harm more likely: unstable workflows, recurring friction, weak signals, poorly supported adaptation, and changes in system behavior that conventional oversight may not register clearly. From that perspective, patient safety becomes more than a method for investigating failure. It becomes a way of governing risk before failure becomes the event that commands attention.

## Shifting From Causation to Anticipation

Retrospective analysis asks: What went wrong? Anticipatory governance asks: Where is fragility accumulating now? The distinction is not semantic. It reflects a fundamental shift in epistemology.

Traditional patient safety governance is event-triggered. Harm generates inquiry. Inquiry generates corrective action. Stability is inferred in the absence of reported events. Yet complex adaptive systems do not fail suddenly; they drift. Small adaptations accumulate. Workarounds normalize. Performance pressures reconfigure priorities. Over time, the system operates further from its formal design while appearing outwardly stable [1].

This phenomenon, often described as "drift into failure," reveals the limitations of event-driven oversight [1]. By the time a sentinel event occurs, the conditions that made it possible have often been present for months or years.

Anticipatory systems reject the assumption that the absence of harm equals the absence of risk. They treat everyday performance as a source of diagnostic information. Instead of focusing solely on deviations, they examine how care succeeds under constraint [2, 3]. In doing so, they surface the adaptive adjustments that prevent harm and the strain those adjustments conceal.

This perspective reframes human variability. Within reactive paradigms, variability is treated primarily as risk to be constrained. Within anticipatory paradigms, variability is understood as both stabilizing and destabilizing [2]. Clinicians routinely adapt to compensate for poorly aligned workflows, cognitive overload, interface friction, and environmental constraints. These adaptations are often heroic. When success depends on continuous compensation, the system is not robust. It is fragile but buffered [3].

Anticipatory governance seeks to identify fragility before buffering capacity is exhausted. It requires institutional mechanisms capable of detecting weak signals: minor inefficiencies, recurring clarifications, near-miss patterns, documentation burden spikes, workflow bottlenecks, patient confusion, and fatigue-related performance variability [4]. These signals rarely appear dramatic. Their importance lies in aggregation.

The shift from causation to anticipation, therefore, requires expanding the object of inquiry. The question is no longer confined to discrete adverse events. It includes emerging conditions, cumulative strain, and misalignments between formal policy and lived practice. In this framing, patient safety becomes prospective.

## Designing for Reliability: Operationalizing Proactive Safety

If anticipation is the shift, then reliability is its operational expression. Healthcare has historically treated reliability as the byproduct of compliance. If protocols are followed, if checklists are leveraged and completed, and if training is delivered, reliability is presumed to follow. This assumption rests on a mechanistic model of performance: standardize inputs and outputs will stabilize [3].

But in complex adaptive systems, standardization alone does not guarantee stability. Standardization reduces variation in controlled domains; it does not eliminate variation in the real world. Healthcare environmental conditions introduce pressure, interruption, ambiguity, and competing priorities. Reliability, therefore, cannot be assumed; it must be demonstrated under stress. This is where proactive patient safety diverges most clearly from retrospective governance.

Retrospective governance waits for system failure to reveal fragility. Proactive governance deliberately exposes fragility. Structured stress testing embodies this philosophy. When workflows are simulated under realistic conditions before implementation, hidden dependencies surface. Equipment placement that appears efficient in blueprint form may impede coordination in motion. Communication channels that appear clear in policy may fracture under time compression. Environmental design may constrain movement during surge conditions. These are not rare defects; they are structural blind spots that only become visible when the system is placed under strain [5].

The principle is deceptively simple: systems behave differently under load. Healthcare often discovers this truth through crisis. Proactive systems choose to discover it through design.

Prospective hazard analysis similarly shifts the timeline of learning. Rather than reconstructing failure after patient harm, organizations model where failure is likely to emerge. This reframes patient safety from forensic activity to anticipatory engineering. It treats risk as a structural property of system configuration rather than an episodic deviation.

Yet stress testing and hazard modeling alone are insufficient if they rely solely on formal representations of work. Policies describe work-as-imagined. Reliability depends on work-as-done. Human-centered inquiry makes this distinction visible. Observational methods reveal how clinicians actually navigate constraints, how documentation competes with patient interaction, how electronic interfaces shape cognitive flow, and how informal coordination compensates for design gaps [6]. These compensations often prevent immediate harm… but they also signal latent misalignment.

Weak signals are particularly instructive. Minor delays, repeated clarifications, cognitive interruptions, navigation friction: each may appear inconsequential in isolation. Aggregated, they indicate systemic strain. Journey mapping approaches have demonstrated that these weak signals often precede measurable adverse outcomes [7]. What organizations classify as noise frequently constitutes early warning.

Design thinking methodologies reinforce this insight by reframing problem definition itself. Instead of beginning with predefined improvement targets, they begin with an inquiry into lived experience [8]. The goal is not creative ideation for its own sake. It is diagnostic precision. If the problem is misdefined, the intervention will optimize the wrong variable.

Reliability, therefore, is not achieved by refining corrective actions alone. It is achieved by validating system performance under realistic variation before exposure to irreversible consequence. This represents a structural departure from traditional safety governance.

Traditional governance assumes sufficiency once policy is written and training is delivered. Proactive governance assumes insufficiency until performance has been demonstrated. The difference is philosophical as much as procedural. It replaces the presumption of correctness with the discipline of interrogation. For instance, policies assume compliance equals patient safety. Proactive systems ask whether compliance produces reliability under stress. The distinction is consequential.

Consider health information technology. Electronic systems are often implemented based on functional adequacy. Does the system allow order entry, documentation, and reconciliation? Yet usability research reveals that interface design can introduce safety risk independent of clinical knowledge [6]. Alert overload, ambiguous display hierarchy, and fragmented navigation pathways alter cognition. The system shapes human performance.

When reliability is treated as an emergent property of socio-technical interaction rather than procedural adherence, design becomes central to patient safety. The question shifts from "Did the clinician follow protocol?" to "Was the system designed to support correct performance under constraint?"

Proactive reliability requires layered mechanisms:

- Continuous detection of weak signals
- Structured stress testing before full-scale deployment
- Iterative prototyping under realistic variation
- Ongoing validation rather than one-time implementation

There is also a governance implication. When proactive mechanisms are embedded upstream, the organization reduces its dependence on heroics downstream. It moves from rewarding individuals who compensate for poor design to redesigning systems so compensation is unnecessary. Reliability, in this framing, is not the absence of failure but rather the absence of preventable fragility.

## Preconditions for Proactive Safety Maturity

Organizations sometimes approach anticipatory frameworks as if they were technical upgrades: adopt a new assessment tool, implement a new reporting platform, introduce a new methodology. Yet proactive patient safety is not a method layered onto an unchanged system. It is a shift in institutional posture. Without structural and cultural alignment, proactive mechanisms collapse into symbolic compliance.

The first precondition is psychological safety. Anticipatory systems depend on the surfacing of weak signals. Weak signals are fragile. They are often ambiguous, socially risky, and easy to dismiss. If frontline staff perceive that identifying fragility will invite scrutiny or reputational harm, signals will remain unvoiced. Silence will be misinterpreted as stability.

Safety culture research consistently demonstrates that reporting behavior reflects trust more than event frequency [9]. In proactive systems, reporting is not merely about patient safety event counts; it is about relational transparency. Staff must believe that surfacing design vulnerability will lead to redesign rather than blame. Without this belief, anticipatory governance is epistemically blind.

But psychological safety alone is insufficient.

Proactive patient safety requires systems literacy. The ability to perceive interdependencies, feedback loops, and nonlinear effects is not intuitive; it must be cultivated. Research linking systems thinking competencies with patient safety performance underscores that anticipatory capacity correlates with cognitive orientation [10]. When professionals are trained primarily to optimize local tasks without visibility into broader system dynamics, they may inadvertently reinforce drift while believing they are improving performance.

Systems literacy transforms how risk is perceived. Instead of asking, "Did I complete the required step?" professionals begin asking, "How does this step interact with upstream and downstream processes?" This changes the accountability lens from individual task completion to collective system integrity.

The third precondition concerns human performance safeguards. Healthcare has historically relied on professional resilience as a stabilizing force. Extended work hours, irregular schedules, cognitive overload, and environmental distractions are often normalized. Yet, fatigue science suggests that performance degradation under such conditions is predictable rather than exceptional [11]. Treating fatigue as an individual failing obscures its structural origins.

Proactive governance reframes human variability as a design parameter. If reliability depends on sustained attention and cognitive capacity, then scheduling, staffing, and workload distribution become patient safety interventions, not human resources considerations. Systems that require continuous heroics to maintain performance are brittle.

A fourth precondition concerns equity. Patient safety risk is not distributed evenly. Harm is shaped by language, disability, race, socioeconomic position, digital access, and the social conditions that influence how patients move through systems of care. When safety metrics are aggregated without attention to differences, important forms of vulnerability remain hidden.

Recent work on integrating health equity and patient safety has emphasized that safety systems must examine not only overall harm rates, but also where structural conditions create unequal exposure to risk [12]. In proactive systems, this means asking whose weak signals are least likely to be noticed, whose burden is least visible in standard metrics, and which populations are most affected by fragmented coordination or confusing design.

These preconditions—psychological safety, systems literacy, human performance safeguards, and equity-informed oversight—form the infrastructure of proactive maturity. Importantly, maturity is cumulative. Organizations do not transition abruptly from reactive to anticipatory. They evolve along a continuum.

At an early stage, safety remains largely reactive. Reporting systems focus on events, investigations are triggered by harm, and improvement efforts concentrate on visible breakdowns.

At an intermediate stage, organizations begin to use prospective methods such as simulation, design-based inquiry, or hazard review, but these remain episodic and weakly connected to strategy.

At more mature stages, anticipation becomes structurally embedded. Leadership reviews forward-looking risk alongside retrospective events. Weak signals are treated as meaningful. Prototyping and stress testing precede large-scale change. Workload and fatigue are recognized as safety concerns. Equity considerations enter both measurement and governance.

Maturity is visible not in the absence of adverse events, but in the organization's capacity to detect fragility before events occur. This distinction clarifies an uncomfortable truth: organizations can achieve strong retrospective metrics while remaining structurally fragile. Low event rates do not necessarily indicate resilience; they may indicate successful compensation.

Anticipation is cognitively and politically demanding. It requires allocating attention and resources to risks that have not yet manifested. It challenges short-term performance metrics by privileging long-term stability. It often produces insights that implicate organizational structure rather than frontline execution. This is why proactive patient safety is not simply a technical progression; it's governance.

## The Proactive Patient Safety Continuum

If causation explains the past and anticipation governs the future, then the task before healthcare is not methodological substitution but architectural integration.

Retrospective investigation remains indispensable. It reveals where harm has crystallized and where system defenses have failed. But when investigation becomes the dominant mode of safety governance, the organization becomes dependent on failure as its primary teacher. The proactive safety continuum breaks this dependency.

At one end of the continuum lies retrospective analysis: root cause investigations, morbidity and mortality conferences, sentinel event reviews. These mechanisms clarify breakdowns and expose latent conditions after harm has occurred.

Moving upstream, prospective hazard identification interrogates system configuration before exposure. Structured stress testing, simulation-based systems validation, and workflow modeling reveal fragility under controlled strain [5]. Instead of learning from catastrophe, organizations learn from rehearsal.

Further upstream, weak signal detection surfaces drift before it becomes measurable failure. Minor inefficiencies, recurring workarounds, cognitive overload, and navigation friction are early markers of misalignment [6]. In mature systems, such signals are not dismissed as operational noise, but as strategic intelligence.

Running parallel to these detection mechanisms is iterative redesign. Prototypes are tested under realistic variation before scaling. Interventions demonstrate reliability before institutionalization. Design assumptions are interrogated rather than presumed.

Downstream, learning is institutionalized through governance feedback loops. Data informs design. Design informs policy. Policy informs training. Training informs performance. Performance informs further inquiry. The system becomes reflexive. The continuum, therefore, consists of interconnected layers:

- Patient safety event investigation
- Prospective hazard modeling
- Weak signal detection
- Structured stress testing
- Iterative redesign
- Governance feedback integration

When integrated, these layers transform patient safety from episodic to continuous stewardship.

Digital technologies introduce both opportunity and risk within this continuum. Real-time predictive analytics and wearable monitoring systems promise earlier detection of physiologic deterioration and operational strain [13]. Yet, predictive capacity does not eliminate complexity… it simply redistributes it. Algorithms encode assumptions. Alerts alter cognitive flow. Automation can obscure as much as it reveals. Technology must therefore be embedded within human-centered governance rather than treated as a substitute for it.

Resilience engineering provides conceptual coherence to this continuum. The evolution from high-reliability organization theory toward human-centered resilience frameworks reflects recognition that control alone cannot produce safety in complex systems [14]. Adaptive capacity must be cultivated, and feedback and learning must be continuous.

The proactive patient safety continuum embodies this evolution. It reframes patient safety as an ongoing design responsibility distributed across leadership, operations, and frontline practice.

- In reactive systems, safety may be treated as the work of dedicated departments, triggered by reportable events. In proactive systems, safety becomes part of governance and design.
- In reactive systems, institutional response is often demonstrated by issuing policy, updating education, or documenting corrective action. In proactive systems, response must be shown in how the system performs under variation.
- In reactive systems, harm remains the main prompt for learning. In proactive systems, drift, strain, and weak signals begin to work earlier.

This move is demanding because it asks institutions to care about risks that have not yet become dramatic. It asks leaders to value invisible prevention as much as visible crisis response. Yet without this transition, healthcare remains in a repetitive position: learning deeply from yesterday's failure while tomorrow's fragility accumulates in quieter form.

The next step, therefore, is methodological. If anticipatory governance is to function, organizations need reliable ways of surfacing weak signals, making work-as-done visible, and converting insight into redesign. The following chapter turns to that question by examining the design toolkit needed to operationalize proactive patient safety in daily clinical systems.

## Conclusion

A proactive patient safety framework does not eliminate the need for retrospective analysis. Serious events still require careful investigation, accountability, and institutional response. What changes is the timing and scope of learning. Organizations become less dependent on visible breakdown as the first meaningful sign that something in the system requires attention.

That shift carries practical consequences. It changes what leaders monitor, what kinds of evidence they treat as actionable, and how they understand the relationship between adaptation and risk.

Weak signals, structured stress testing, prospective hazard identification, and iterative redesign matter because they make fragility more visible while the system is still functioning. The work of patient safety becomes less episodic and more continuous.

It also becomes more demanding. Anticipatory governance asks institutions to notice patterns that are easier to dismiss than a reportable event, to treat strain as significant before it produces public failure, and to invest in redesign before consequences force recognition. That requires more than a new vocabulary. It requires methods that can make system behavior visible, test assumptions under realistic conditions, and translate emerging insight into action. Without those methods, proactive safety remains persuasive in principle but difficult to sustain in practice.

## References

1. Peerally MF, Carr S, Waring J, Dixon-Woods M. The problem with root cause analysis. BMJ Qual Saf. 2017;26(5):417–22. https://doi.org/10.1136/bmjqs-2016-005511.
2. Young RA, Xiao Y, Fulda KG. Safety-I versus Safety-II: a mixed-methods study revealing the imbalance of approaches in primary care medication safety. J Patient Saf. 2025;21(Suppl 1):S81–8. https://doi.org/10.1097/PTS.0000000000001400.
3. Agency for Healthcare Research and Quality. Understand the science of safety. In: Comprehensive unit-based safety program (CUSP) toolkit. Rockville: AHRQ; 2024. Available from: https://www.ahrq.gov/hai/cusp/modules/index.html.
4. Scanlon MC, Jacobson M. Safety I, Safety II, and new views of safety. PSNet primer. Rockville: Agency for Healthcare Research and Quality; 2025. Available from: https://psnet.ahrq.gov.
5. Hazwani T, Hamam H, Caswell A, Madkhaly A, Al Saif S, Al Hassan Z, et al. Proactive patient safety: enhancing hospital readiness through simulation-based clinical systems testing and healthcare failure mode and effect analysis. Adv Simul. 2024;9(1):26. https://doi.org/10.1186/s41077-024-00298-z.
6. Awad S, Begg R, Loveday T, Baysari MT. Using human centred design and human factors to support a rapid health information technology patient safety response. BMC Health Serv Res. 2025;25:1169. https://doi.org/10.1186/s12913-025-13293-5.
7. Cunha AS, Cordeiro JV, Victorino G. Uncovering "weak signals" through patient journey mapping to inform the future redesign of the medical con-

sultation room. BMC Health Serv Res. 2026;26:227. https://doi.org/10.1186/s12913-026-14037-9.
8. Del-Valle Quintana L, Sichieri K, Secoli S. Design thinking and its use to promote patient safety: a scoping review. J Healthc Qual Res. 2025;40(4):101140. https://doi.org/10.1016/j.jhqr.2025.101140.
9. Murray J, Sorra J, Gale B, Mossburg S. Ensuring patient and workforce safety culture in healthcare. PSNet perspective. Rockville: Agency for Healthcare Research and Quality; 2024. Available from: https://psnet.ahrq.gov/perspective/ensuring-patient-and-workforce-safety-culture-healthcare.
10. Atalla ADG, Bahr RRR, El-Sayed AAI. Exploring the hidden synergy between system thinking and patient safety competencies among critical care nurses: a cross-sectional study. BMC Nurs. 2025;24:114. https://doi.org/10.1186/s12912-025-02717-6.
11. Fox S, Dall'Ora C, Young M. Fatigue risk management in healthcare: a scoping literature review. Int J Nurs Stud. 2026;174:105282. https://doi.org/10.1016/j.ijnurstu.2025.105282.
12. Tsuei J, Bandini JI, Thomas AD, James KF, Etchegaray JM, Schulson L. A systems-based framework for integrating health equity and patient safety. Jt Comm J Qual Patient Saf. 2025;51(7–8):498–506. https://doi.org/10.1016/j.jcjq.2025.04.005.
13. Mahajan A, Heydari K, Powell D. Wearable AI to enhance patient safety and clinical decision-making. NPJ Digit Med. 2025;8:176. https://doi.org/10.1038/s41746-025-01554-w.
14. Guttman O, Konwinski LM, Moses J, Henwood PC. From HRO to HRE: human-centered resilience engineering as an evolving framework for patient safety management. NEJM Catal Innov Care Deliv. 2025;7(1):1–19. https://doi.org/10.1056/CAT.25.0162.

# The Design Toolkit for Proactive Patient Safety

# 8

## Introduction

Proactive patient safety is compelling at the level of principle. Concepts such as anticipatory governance, weak signal detection, resilience, and structured stress testing offer a coherent account of how healthcare organizations might move beyond event-triggered learning. Yet concepts do not alter practice by themselves. They become consequential only when organizations have practical ways to observe system behavior, interpret emerging fragility, and redesign care processes before harm occurs.

Most patient safety professionals are deeply experienced in retrospective investigation, compliance review, audit, and performance monitoring. They know how to analyze adverse events, document corrective action, and respond to regulatory expectations. What is less consistently available are practical methods for observing work-as-done, identifying latent strain, reframing risk before harm becomes visible, and testing interventions under real variation. The intellectual case for anticipatory safety may already be understood. The operational methods often are not.

Design tools are relevant because they address that gap. The phrase design thinking sometimes generates skepticism in clinical settings, particularly when patient safety is at stake. It may evoke workshop culture, facilitation techniques, or forms of creativity that appear insufficiently rigorous for a field grounded in ethics,


K. Rasmussen, *Rethinking Patient Safety*,
https://doi.org/10.1007/978-3-032-26054-3_8

reliability, and accountability. That skepticism is understandable when design is used superficially. The issue is not the term. It is the standard of application.

Used with discipline, design methods offer structured ways of working within complexity. They help organizations surface drift before it becomes reportable harm, identify compensatory behaviors that conceal fragility, and test assumptions before those assumptions are embedded in policy or technology. In that sense, the methods are not ancillary to safety science. They are one way of extending it into conditions where workflow, cognition, environment, and lived experience all matter at once.

Healthcare systems are layered and interdependent. Policies interact with workflows. Technology shapes cognition. Staffing levels influence decision quality. Equity shapes exposure to risk. Hazards emerge from misalignment across these layers rather than from isolated points of failure. Traditional improvement tools perform well when the problem is stable and clearly defined. They are less effective when the problem itself is poorly understood or when the intervention reshapes the system in unpredictable ways.

The tools that follow are intended for that purpose. Some help make drift visible in daily work. Others support problem framing, bounded testing, or the translation of local insight into broader institutional learning. Their value lies less in novelty than in whether they allow organizations to see more clearly, test more carefully, and act before fragility becomes public failure.

## Maintaining Methodological Integrity

Design methods do not automatically produce insight. They can clarify complexity or obscure it. Their value depends less on the tool selected and more on the posture with which it is applied.

In environments where patient harm is at stake, methodological credibility cannot be assumed. Tools that lack rigor weaken trust rather than strengthen safety. For design methods to contribute meaningfully to patient safety, they must be applied with discipline, ethical awareness, and structural integration. The guardrails that follow define the conditions under which this toolkit reinforces safety architecture rather than producing surface-level activity:

**1. Begin with Reality, Not Representation**

Healthcare organizations possess detailed representations of work: policies, workflows, protocols, escalation pathways, competency checklists, and audit dashboards. These representations are necessary, but they are not sufficient.

Design work begins in lived conditions. Policies describe work-as-imagined. Safety performance unfolds within work-as-done. The gap between the two is not an anomaly; it is structural. Clinicians adapt continuously to time pressure, cognitive load, technology friction, and resource constraints. These adaptations are often invisible in formal documentation.

When design tools are applied to representations alone, they reinforce institutional assumptions. Applied to reality, they surface drift. This requires deliberate exposure to the environment under both normal and stressed conditions. Observing during peak census, shift transitions, staffing variability, or electronic downtime reveals vulnerabilities that controlled settings conceal. Without that grounding, redesign efforts may optimize a formal process that has only partial correspondence to the work itself.

**2. Treat Experience as Operational Data**

Clinical environments often categorize frustration, confusion, and workaround behavior as soft signals. Yet these experiences reflect measurable system strain. When documentation demands crowd out patient interaction or alerts are routinely overridden, the system is communicating.

Design methods convert lived experience into structured data. Cognitive burden, emotional escalation, clarification frequency, and workaround dependence can be mapped, categorized, and analyzed. Treated rigorously, experiential insight becomes a leading indicator of fragility.

This guardrail protects against superficial empathy exercises. The objective is not storytelling for its own sake; it's diagnostic precision. Experience becomes actionable when translated into observable patterns and linked to system configuration.

**3. Make Assumptions Explicit Before Designing Solutions**

Healthcare improvement initiatives often move quickly from problem recognition to intervention. That speed is understandable, especially when the issue is visible and the pressure to act is high. It also creates risk. Organizations frequently build solutions on assumptions that have never been articulated, much less tested.

Common examples include assumptions that staff have time for the added step, that an alert will be noticed and interpreted correctly, that patients understand instructions as written, or that training will compensate for poor system fit. Design methods slow this movement just enough to surface such assumptions. Once named, they can be tested.

This is one of the central contributions of the toolkit. It prevents organizations from formalizing interventions whose success depends on conditions that are not actually present in practice.

**4. Test Under Variation, Not Under Ideal Conditions**

Healthcare systems rarely operate under stable conditions. Interventions that perform well only under ideal circumstances carry hidden vulnerability. A core guardrail of this toolkit is therefore exposure to variation before scale. Workflows must be tested during surge. Interfaces should be evaluated amid interruption. Escalation pathways require exercise under cognitive overload. Equity implications must be examined across differences in language, literacy, and access.

Performance observed in calm conditions does not predict behavior under strain. Testing across variation grounds safety redesign in demonstrated reliability rather than assumed stability.

**5. Distinguish Between Artifact Production and System Learning**

Design processes generate visible artifacts: maps, personas, journey diagrams, prototypes, and reframed problem statements. These outputs can create a persuasive sense of movement without producing structural change. When an empathy exercise does not influence staffing decisions or a journey map fails to inform resource allocation, the work remains symbolic rather than systemic.

Patient safety depends on institutional learning, not artifact production. This guardrail requires that design outputs be translated into governance decisions. Each tool in this chapter includes guidance on how its results should inform policy revision, resource allocation, performance measurement, or structural redesign. Without such integration, design activity remains adjacent to safety architecture rather than embedded within it.

**6. Preserve Ethical Discipline**

Design in patient safety carries ethical weight. Observation occurs in environments where privacy, dignity, and vulnerability are present. Prototyping unfolds in systems where unintended consequences are not theoretical. Staff participation reflects power dynamics that must be acknowledged. Equity analysis involves real communities whose experiences cannot be treated as abstract inputs.

For that reason, design in this context is not a neutral inquiry. It is a structured intervention within morally consequential systems. Deliberate reflection, transparent communication, and explicit risk review are necessary at every stage. The pursuit of innovation cannot override the discipline required to protect those the system is meant to serve.

These guardrails establish the posture from which the toolkit should be used. Once that posture is in place, the first substantive task is visibility. Drift cannot be addressed if it remains unobserved.

## Making Drift Visible in Clinical Systems

Anticipatory patient safety begins with disciplined visibility. Drift cannot be corrected if it remains unexamined. In complex clinical systems, fragility rarely appears as a dramatic breakdown. It accumulates incrementally through adaptation, workaround, and rising cognitive demand. The task of discovery is to render that accumulation visible before it crystallizes into harm.

Discovery is not an exercise in confirmation. It challenges institutional representations of how work is presumed to occur. Policies, dashboards, and compliance reports describe intended structure; they do not capture the lived negotiations through which care is actually delivered. Contemporary safety scholarship has emphasized this distinction between work-as-imagined and work-as-done as central to understanding system performance [1, 2]. Visibility, therefore, requires empirical engagement with real conditions.

## Observing Work-as-Done in Clinical Systems

Patient safety has traditionally been organized around event investigation. Work-as-done observation changes the temporal sequence. Rather than waiting until a reportable event has occurred, the organization studies how care is currently being sustained and where that performance is becoming increasingly dependent on adaptation.

**Definition** Contextual observation is a structured method for examining work-as-done within real clinical environments. It involves a systematic, in situ study of how tasks are performed under routine and stressed conditions, with explicit attention to adaptation, workaround behavior, cognitive load, and environmental constraint. Unlike retrospective investigation, contextual observation is prospective and diagnostic. Its purpose is to identify emerging fragility and compensatory patterns before measurable harm occurs.

Policies, protocols, and escalation pathways describe work-as-imagined. Clinical care unfolds as work-as-done [3]. The distinction between the two is central to contemporary safety science [1, 2]. Drift emerges within the space separating representation from reality. Observation brings that space into view.

Clinicians routinely adjust sequencing, timing, and communication patterns in response to workload, cognitive demand, environmental constraint, and technology friction. Documentation may be deferred to preserve patient interaction. Informal clarification loops may replace formal escalation channels. Alerts may be preemptively overridden when they are perceived as misaligned with clinical context. Human factors research has demonstrated that these behaviors are rational responses to design conditions rather than isolated lapses [4].

Adaptation is frequently protective. Resilience engineering scholarship emphasizes that adaptive capacity enables systems to function under variability [5]. The question for anticipatory safety is not whether adaptation occurs, but whether adaptation has become the system's primary stabilizing mechanism. When reliability depends on informal coordination, memory, vigilance, or endurance rather than structural alignment, fragility is accumulating.

Observation should therefore focus on markers of strain. These may include:

- Recurring pauses or hesitations
- Informal clarification loops
- Tasks completed out of sequence
- Interruptions and recovery strategies
- Signals of cognitive overload
- Workarounds that bypass formal process
- Environmental constraints shaping behavior

Each indicator may appear minor in isolation. However, their significance lies in repetition and aggregation.

Observation must also extend beyond stable conditions. Performance shifts under surge, staffing variability, technology downtime, and differences in experience level. Simulation-based systems testing has shown that system behavior under load reveals vulnerabilities not visible during equilibrium [6]. Reliability observed in calm conditions offers limited assurance under strain.

Methodological discipline distinguishes contextual observation from anecdote. Teams should document intended workflow alongside observed workflow, noting where adaptation occurs and why. Each adaptation should be examined in relation to the constraint prompting it and the risk it mitigates or introduces. Patterns should be tracked across time and across roles rather than attributed to individual behavior. Structured comparison between representation and lived execution transforms observation from narrative into analyzable data.

Interpretation requires restraint. Not all deviations increase risk. Some adaptations compensate for design gaps and prevent harm. Safety-II scholarship underscores that understanding why work succeeds is as important as understanding why it fails [1–3]. The analytical task is to distinguish adaptive resilience from compensatory fragility. If an adaptation reduces workload without introducing new risk, it may reflect healthy flexibility. If it shifts burden, increases cognitive demand, or depends on memory under pressure, it may signal drift.

When conducted rigorously, contextual observation recalibrates governance perception. Apparent noncompliance may reflect interface ambiguity. Recurrent clarification may reveal communication design flaws. Persistent workaround patterns may indicate structural misalignment rather than individual error. Weak signal research suggests that such patterns frequently precede measurable adverse outcomes [7]. Observation therefore functions as an early warning.

Contextual observation is not exploratory curiosity. It recalibrates how the organization understands the relationship between formal process and actual performance. Once this is visible, the analysis can widen from discrete tasks to the broader pathways through which patients and staff move.

## Mapping Experience and System Interactions Across Care

Observation reveals local adaptation. Mapping shows how those local adjustments accumulate across transitions, roles, and episodes of care. In patient safety, this is critical because fragility often emerges not within a single step, but across the interfaces that connect steps together.

## Journey Mapping in Patient Safety Context

A patient's experience of care is rarely contained within one interaction. It unfolds across a sequence of touchpoints, transitions, decisions, and delays. At each point, information may be transferred, lost, repeated, or misunderstood. Risk frequently accumulates in these interfaces.

**Definition** Patient journey mapping is a structured method for visually representing the sequence of interactions, decisions, transitions, and experiences that constitute an episode of care as lived by a defined individual or group. Unlike workflow diagrams, which depict formal process steps, journey maps capture how those steps are experienced, including perceptions, emotions, uncertainty, cognitive burden, and informal adaptations. In patient safety applications, journey mapping identifies recurring friction, misalignment, and strain that may signal emerging risk.

Journey mapping differs fundamentally from workflow mapping. Workflow diagrams describe how tasks are intended to proceed within an organization. Journey maps describe how those tasks are experienced by a person moving through the system. The distinction is not semantic. It shifts the unit of analysis from institutional process to lived experience.

In practice, a journey map traces an individual's trajectory across an episode of care and overlays several layers of information:

- Key touchpoints and transitions
- Actions taken or required
- Information exchanged
- Decisions encountered
- Points of confusion or delay
- Emotional response or perceived burden

Emotional trajectory is included as data. Human factors research has long recognized that subjective states such as frustration and mental effort are measurable components of cognitive workload [8]. In clinical environments, fluctuations in stress and cognitive load influence attention, working memory, and decision reliability [9]. Sustained emotional strain, including burnout, further degrades performance and increases vulnerability to error [10]. Interpreted through this lens, variation in emotional intensity across a care journey reflects shifts in cognitive demand rather than isolated affect. This logic aligns with cognitive load theory, which emphasizes the relationship between mental effort and performance capacity in medical settings [11].

Weak signal research supports the value of examining such recurring friction. Patterns of repeated clarification, delays at transition points, or patient confusion about next steps often precede measurable adverse events [7]. When aggregated across journeys, these signals shift from anecdote to structural indicator.

Journey mapping applies to any defined actor navigating the system. A family member coordinating discharge, a nurse reconciling medications, or a resident managing overnight cross-cover each traverses a sequence of transitions shaped by system design. What changes is the persona; the analytic logic remains constant.

Effective journey mapping requires:

- A defined persona
- A bounded episode of care
- Observed rather than assumed steps
- Explicit identification of friction and adaptation
- Documentation of cognitive or emotional trajectory
- Synthesis into structural hypotheses

When constructed intentionally, journey maps help organizations identify where risk accumulates across time rather than where it simply becomes visible at the end (Fig. 8.1).

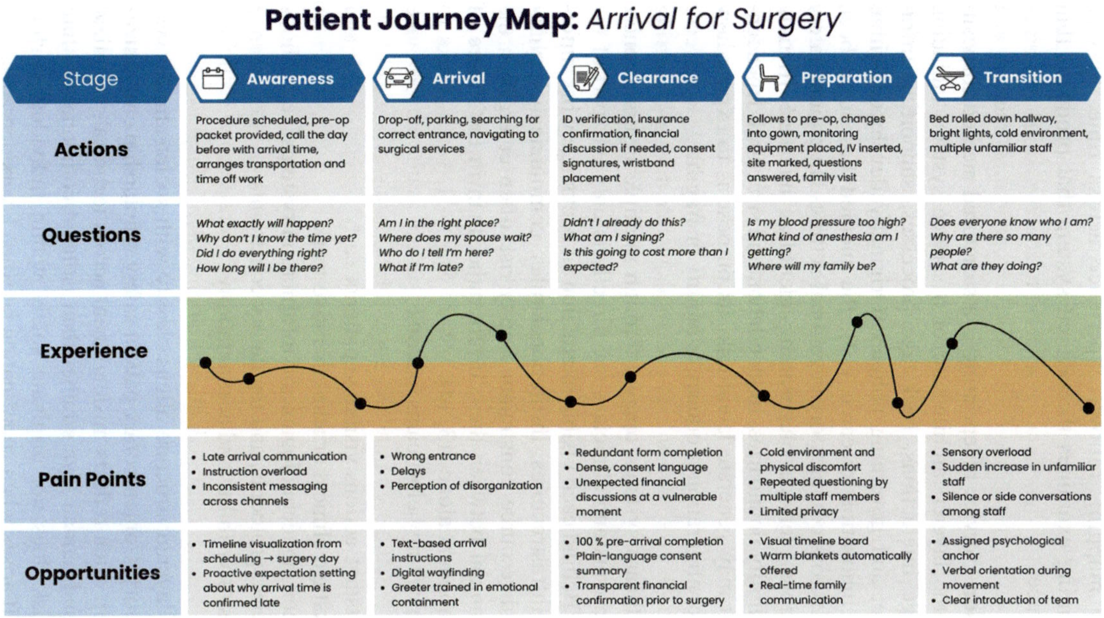


**Fig. 8.1** An example of a patient journey map used for proactive safety analysis. The map illustrates a defined persona moving through sequential care touchpoints across a bounded episode of care

## Service Blueprinting

Journey mapping follows experience across time. Service blueprinting examines the layered system that produces that experience.

**Definition** Service blueprinting is a structured method for visualizing the layered architecture of a service system, including frontstage interactions, backstage processes, supporting infrastructure, and governing policies. Originally developed within service innovation research [12], the method has since been applied across complex organizational settings. In patient safety applications, service blueprinting identifies interface friction, responsibility boundaries, hidden labor, and structural dependencies that may generate latent risk. Its purpose is to expose how system configuration produces reliability or fragility.

Healthcare systems operate through multiple layers at once. What patients and clinicians see directly is only one part of the system. Behind each visible interaction sit backstage work, information infrastructures, institutional rules, communication channels, and resource constraints. Safety risk often emerges in the misalignment between these layers rather than in the failure of one component alone [13, 14].

Blueprinting helps teams examine:

- Frontstage actions visible to patients
- Backstage clinical or administrative work
- Supporting technologies and information systems
- Policies, protocols, and regulatory constraints
- Lines of visibility and accountability

This layered structure aligns closely with sociotechnical systems theory. Contemporary patient safety scholarship emphasizes that harm often reflects misalignment across technical, organizational, and human layers rather than isolated component failure [13]. Risk does not originate solely within individual performance. It arises when coordination between layers degrades.

In patient safety contexts, blueprinting reveals where experience and infrastructure diverge. A patient may experience a delay at discharge, while backstage coordination between pharmacy, nursing, and insurance verification is fragmented. A clinician may appear slow in documentation, while the electronic health record imposes navigation burdens that fragment attention. A resident may hesitate during escalation, while supervision structures create ambiguity in authority.

Human-centered design research demonstrates that interface architecture influences cognition, attention allocation, and decision-making independent of professional competence [4]. Service blueprinting situates these interface dynamics within the broader system configuration rather than isolating them as usability complaints.

Several structural patterns frequently emerge in blueprint analysis:

- Hidden labor becomes visible. Work performed informally to maintain reliability often resides backstage and remains unrecognized in formal process descriptions. When reliability depends on invisible coordination, fragility accumulates.
- Responsibility boundaries clarify points of vulnerability. When accountability crosses layers without explicit reinforcement, coordination relies on memory and vigilance rather than structure.
- Interface congestion appears where multiple layers intersect. Technology, policy, and clinical judgment may converge at a single decision point, increasing cognitive stacking.
- Feedback pathways reveal whether outcomes inform upstream design. When performance data fails to reshape infrastructure, drift persists.

Simulation-based systems testing has demonstrated that service configuration behaves differently under load [6]. A blueprint constructed under routine conditions may conceal stress fractures that appear during a surge. Anticipatory blueprinting, therefore, incorporates variation, documenting how layer interactions shift when staffing fluctuates, census rises, or digital systems degrade.

Service blueprinting also strengthens equity analysis. By visualizing layers of infrastructure and policy, it becomes possible to identify where access barriers are embedded structurally rather than individually. Digital portals, transportation dependencies, insurance verification processes, and language services can be examined not as peripheral concerns but as architectural components of safety exposure.

Journey maps and service blueprints are most powerful when used together. One shows how the system is lived. The other shows how it is built. Integrated, these tools move patient safety teams from narrative insight to structural diagnosis.

Yet insights and structure do not automatically determine which variable demands intervention. Once friction has been mapped, a more disciplined question emerges: What, precisely, must change?

## Framing the Problem Before Solving It

Contemporary patient safety scholarship emphasizes that outcomes emerge from dynamic interactions among people, tasks, tools, organizational structures, and environmental conditions rather than from isolated components [14]. Without disciplined problem framing, redesign efforts risk addressing symptoms while leaving architecture intact. In complex systems, the way a problem is defined shapes the trajectory of every subsequent intervention. Misalignment at the framing stage propagates downstream, institutionalizing well-intentioned but structurally fragile solutions. Before the redesign begins, assumptions must be surfaced and examined.

Assumption mapping introduces methodological restraint at precisely this juncture. Instead of moving directly from identified friction to intervention, teams articulate the conditions that must hold true for a proposed change to produce reliable performance. These conditions often concern workload capacity, cognitive bandwidth, technological stability, authority gradients, coordination reliability, or equity access. When left implicit, such assumptions function as hidden dependencies embedded within the system.

The SEIPS 3.0 framework reinforces why this discipline is essential. It conceptualizes healthcare work as the product of interacting system elements whose alignment determines performance and safety [14]. An electronic alert assumes attentional availability and interpretive clarity. A revised discharge protocol assumes language comprehension, stable follow-up access, and cognitive readiness at the moment of transition. Each assumption exists within a broader configuration of constraints. If that configuration cannot sustain the intervention under variation, reliability erodes despite formal compliance.

Implementation science further demonstrates that intervention success is context-dependent rather than intrinsic [14]. Adaptation is not a deviation from fidelity but a recognition that systems vary in capacity and structure. Assumption mapping aligns with this insight by reframing redesign as hypothesis generation rather than declarative correction. The central question shifts from "What should we implement?" to "Under what contextual conditions would this intervention perform reliably?"

Cognitive science adds another layer of caution. Performance capacity is finite and sensitive to environmental demand and task complexity [11]. Acute stress and sustained strain narrow attentional bandwidth and working memory, altering decision reliability [10, 14]. When interventions increase cognitive burden without structural support, they amplify the fragility they aim to mitigate. By explicitly articulating assumptions about capacity, attention, and coordination, organizations surface epistemic risk alongside technical risk.

Assumption mapping therefore functions as a bridge between discovery and validation. It disciplines governance conversation by shifting evaluation from endorsement of ideas to interrogation of premises. What evidence supports the underlying assumptions? What variation might destabilize them? Which system elements have not yet been stress-tested? This posture replaces institutional confidence with structured inquiry, aligning safety redesign with anticipatory governance rather than reactive correction.

Importantly, assumption mapping does not delay action indefinitely. It clarifies which assumptions require validation prior to scale and which can be tested through limited deployment or simulation. Some propositions will prove robust across contexts; others will expose structural dependencies that require redesign before implementation. By converting belief into a testable hypothesis, the organization reduces both operational and epistemic fragility.

Yet hypotheses remain provisional until exposed to operational reality. Even well-framed interventions can destabilize when introduced into live systems characterized by constraint and variability. Framing establishes disciplined intention; only validation determines whether that intention can withstand the pressures of practice. The next step, therefore, is not additional deliberation but structured exposure to variation.

## Validating Change Under Variation

In patient safety work, many interventions move from conceptual agreement to institutional deployment without structured exposure to operational variability. Policy is approved, training is delivered, compliance metrics are defined, and implementation is declared complete. What remains uncertain is whether the intervention performs reliably when introduced into the layered, dynamic conditions of clinical practice. Validation addresses that uncertainty.

Within this toolkit, validation refers to the deliberate testing of an intervention under bounded but realistic conditions before full institutionalization. The objective is not innovation for its own sake. It is disciplined exposure to constraint. A proposed change is placed within the environments in which it must ultimately function and observed for stability, strain, and unintended consequence.

Systems engineering research emphasizes that performance emerges from interaction among people, tasks, tools, and organizational context rather than from any single component [14]. An intervention that appears stable in isolation may behave differently once introduced into existing workflows, authority structures, digital interfaces, and workload pressures. Validation therefore examines interactional effects rather than theoretical coherence.

Bounded prototyping provides one mechanism for this examination. A prototype may involve limited rollout within a single unit, simulated enactment during peak conditions, or structured rehearsal of escalation pathways under time compression. The scale remains intentionally constrained. The purpose is not to achieve immediate performance optimization but to surface vulnerabilities while consequences remain manageable.

Simulation-based clinical systems testing literature demonstrates that structural weaknesses frequently emerge only under load [6]. Communication pathways that appear sufficient under routine census may fracture during a surge. Decision thresholds may shift when cognitive demand increases. Validation leverages this principle by introducing controlled stress prior to scale.

Explicit criteria must guide evaluation. Without predefined indicators of reliability and strain, testing becomes anecdotal and vulnerable to confirmation bias. Measures may include variation in completion time, escalation latency, alert override frequency, documentation burden, coordination breakdowns, or differential impact across patient groups. Where appropriate, stratified analysis should assess whether performance stability holds across language, literacy, or access differences.

Digital interventions require particular scrutiny. Interface modifications alter navigation patterns, information hierarchy, and attentional distribution. Human factors research has demonstrated that subtle design changes can influence decision-making behavior independent of clinical knowledge [4]. Validation examines not only whether a feature functions technically but also whether it supports cognitive flow under interruption and competing demand.

Importantly, validation is iterative rather than singular. Early performance may reflect novelty effects rather than sustained reliability. As contextual pressures shift, previously stable interventions may degrade. Iterative cycles allow teams to observe whether performance stabilizes across variation or whether fragility reappears under new conditions.

Validation does not seek perfection. It seeks evidence of resilience. An intervention need not eliminate variability to be viable, but it must demonstrate that variability does not escalate into predictable failure when conditions change. When failure emerges within bounded testing, it becomes information rather than harm. Structural dependencies are revealed before institutional commitment amplifies consequences. The organization learns under containment rather than through adverse events.

Validation therefore completes the movement initiated in discovery. Visibility exposed drift. Framing clarified assumptions. Validation determines whether the proposed redesign can withstand the realities of practice.

The final step is integration: ensuring that what has been learned through disciplined testing reshapes governance, resource allocation, and oversight rather than remaining localized knowledge.

## Translating Insight into Anticipatory Learning

Observation, mapping, reframing, and validation generate knowledge. That knowledge improves patient safety only if it changes how the organization understands and governs its own system.

This is one of the central challenges in proactive safety work. Design inquiry often produces rich local insight, but that insight may remain contained within the project that generated it. A team may discover that discharge reliability depends on informal nursing work not represented in process design. Another may find that escalation delays are caused by unclear authority boundaries rather than by a knowledge deficit. Unless such findings enter governance, resource decisions, or institutional standards, they remain isolated improvements rather than elements of organizational learning.

Learning health system literature is useful here because it treats frontline experience, operational data, and redesign as part of a continuous cycle rather than a series of disconnected projects

[15]. In that model, design tools do not sit outside governance. They provide one route through which governance gains access to system behavior that conventional dashboards may not detect.

For this to happen, design outputs must be translated. A journey map may need to become a staffing or communication redesign decision. A prototype failure may need to influence technology governance. An insight about burden may need to enter operational planning. Without this translation, the toolkit produces local intelligence without institutional consequence.

That final step is what turns design inquiry into anticipatory learning. The organization moves from seeing weak signals to incorporating them into how it plans, allocates, and redesigns. The purpose of the toolkit is therefore not simply to enrich understanding. It is to strengthen the institution's capacity to act upstream.

## Conclusion

The value of a design toolkit in patient safety lies in what it allows organizations to do earlier and with greater precision. Observation makes drift more visible. Mapping shows where strain accumulates across time, roles, and settings. Reframing prevents premature closure around familiar explanations. Validation tests whether a proposed response can hold under the conditions that will actually shape its use. Taken together, these methods do not replace established safety practices. They extend what those practices are able to see.

That extension matters because anticipatory safety depends on more than intent. Organizations may endorse upstream thinking and still remain largely reactive if they lack practical ways to identify fragility before it produces visible harm. A toolkit of this kind does not solve that problem by itself, but it provides a more workable bridge between abstract commitment and operational practice.

Its significance also depends on whether the resulting insight travels. If observations remain local, if prototypes remain disconnected from governance, or if burden becomes visible without altering decisions about workflow, staffing, or technology, the work remains incomplete. These methods are most useful when they feed institutional learning rather than ending as project artifacts. Used with discipline, they help organizations examine the conditions under which care is actually being delivered and act while those conditions are still modifiable.

## References

1. Scanlon MC, Jacobson M. Safety I, Safety II, and new views of safety. PSNet primer. Agency for Healthcare Research and Quality; 2025. Available from: https://psnet.ahrq.gov.
2. Young RA, Xiao Y, Fulda KG. Safety-I versus Safety-II: a mixed-methods study revealing the imbalance of approaches in primary care medication safety. J Patient Saf. 2025;21(Suppl 1):S81–8. https://doi.org/10.1097/PTS.0000000000001259.
3. Hollnagel E. Safety-I and Safety-II: the past and future of safety management. Farnham: Ashgate Publishing; 2014.
4. Awad S, Begg R, Loveday T, Baysari MT. Using human centred design and human factors to support a rapid health information technology patient safety response. BMC Health Serv Res. 2025;25:1169. https://doi.org/10.1186/s12913-025-13293-5.
5. Guttman O, Konwinski LM, Moses J, Henwood PC. From HRO to HRE: human-centered resilience engineering as an evolving framework for patient safety management. NEJM Catal Innov Care Deliv. 2025;7(1):1–19. https://doi.org/10.1056/CAT.25.0162.
6. Hazwani T, Hamam H, Caswell A, Madkhaly A, Al Saif S, Al Hassan Z, et al. Proactive patient safety: enhancing hospital readiness through simulation-based clinical systems testing and healthcare failure mode and effect analysis. Adv Simul. 2024;9(1):26. https://doi.org/10.1186/s41077-024-00298-z.
7. Cunha AS, Cordeiro JV, Victorino G. Uncovering "weak signals" through patient journey mapping to inform the future redesign of the medical consultation room. BMC Health Serv Res. 2026;26:227. https://doi.org/10.1186/s12913-026-14037-9.
8. Hart SG, Staveland LE. Development of NASA-TLX (Task Load Index): results of empirical and theoretical research. In: Hancock PA, Meshkati N, editors. Human mental workload. Amsterdam: North-Holland; 1988. p. 139–83.
9. Russ SJ, Morrison I, Bell C, Morse JC, Mackenzie RK, Johnston MK. Relationship between acute stress and clinical performance in med-

ical students: a pilot simulation study. BMJ Simul Technol Enhanc Learn. 2018;4(4):171–8. https://doi.org/10.1136/bmjstel-2017-000247.
10. West CP, Dyrbye LN, Shanafelt TD. Physician burnout: contributors, consequences and solutions. J Intern Med. 2018;283(6):516–29. https://doi.org/10.1111/joim.12752.
11. Young JQ, Van Merriënboer J, Durning S, Ten Cate O. Cognitive load theory: implications for medical education. Med Educ. 2014;48(3):225–34. https://doi.org/10.1111/medu.12373.
12. Bitner MJ, Ostrom AL, Morgan FN. Service blueprinting: a practical technique for service innovation. J Serv Res. 2008;8(1):66–94. https://doi.org/10.1177/1094670505281501.
13. Papoutsi C, Reed JE, Marston C, Lewis R, Majeed A, Bell D. Patient safety and the sociotechnical perspective: past, present, and future. BMJ Qual Saf. 2020;29(5):419–25. https://doi.org/10.1136/bmjqs-2019-009485.
14. Carayon P, Wooldridge A, Hoonakker P, Hundt AS, Kelly MM. SEIPS 3.0: human-centered design of the patient journey for patient safety. Appl Ergon. 2020;84:103033. https://doi.org/10.1016/j.apergo.2019.103033.
15. Platt JE, Raj M, Wienroth M, McGowan ML. Embedding a learning health system approach within healthcare organizations. Learn Health Syst. 2022;6(2):e10288. https://doi.org/10.1002/lrh2.10288.

# Measuring and Sustaining Proactive Patient Safety Systems

# 9

## Introduction

Patient safety measurement has long been organized around visible harm. Rates of infection, falls, medication errors, pressure injuries, and other adverse outcomes remain central to how healthcare organizations assess safety performance. These measures are important. They show where patients have been harmed, where systems have failed conspicuously, and where accountability must be sharpened. They also support benchmarking, reporting, and institutional oversight.

Their limits are equally important. Outcome measures register harm after it has occurred. They say relatively little about the conditions under which that harm was becoming more likely while the system still appeared to function. In complex sociotechnical environments, safety does not deteriorate only at the moment an adverse event becomes visible. Fragility often gathers earlier, in shifts in workflow, growing documentation burden, unstable coordination, repeated workarounds, and forms of adaptation that make care possible while also concealing risk [1, 2].

This raises a more difficult question for proactive safety systems. If organizations want to detect risk before serious harm becomes the main source of evidence, what exactly should they measure? Outcome data remain necessary, but they are not sufficient for that task. Measures are also needed that can make opera-



K. Rasmussen, *Rethinking Patient Safety*,
https://doi.org/10.1007/978-3-032-26054-3_9

tional strain, emerging instability, and changes in system behavior more visible while those conditions are still modifiable.

Safety science has increasingly pointed in this direction. A Safety-II perspective, for example, asks how it succeeds under varying conditions and what those patterns of adaptation reveal about system performance [1, 3]. From that standpoint, measurement cannot be confined to counting bad outcomes after the fact. It must also examine how work is being sustained, where burden is accumulating, and whether redesign efforts are improving the conditions under which safe care is produced.

Measurement therefore serves more than a reporting function. It shapes what the organization is able to notice. It influences which forms of strain become legible, which kinds of adaptation remain hidden, and whether leaders can distinguish between systems that are genuinely becoming safer and systems that are simply absorbing more pressure before failure becomes visible. In proactive patient safety, that broader form of visibility becomes essential.

## Rethinking Patient Safety Measurement

### Lagging Indicators: Learning from Harm

Outcome metrics have historically formed the backbone of patient safety measurement. Rates of hospital-acquired infections, medication errors, diagnostic delays, pressure injuries, and patient falls provide important signals about whether harm has occurred within a healthcare system. These measures support regulatory oversight, benchmarking across institutions, and accountability for patient outcomes.

Lagging indicators play a critical role in identifying patterns of harm. When organizations track these measures consistently, they can detect trends that indicate systemic weaknesses. For example, an increase in central line-associated bloodstream infections may reveal problems in catheter insertion protocols or maintenance procedures. Rising surgical site infection rates may signal breakdowns in sterile technique or perioperative antibiotic administration.

However, lagging indicators share a fundamental limitation: they measure harm only after it has occurred. By the time an adverse event appears in outcome data, the system conditions that enabled it may have been developing for months or even years. Researchers studying complex systems have noted that accidents often represent the final stage of a long process in which small adaptations and misalignments accumulate until system defenses are overwhelmed [2]. As a result, healthcare organizations that rely exclusively on outcome metrics may detect safety problems only after patients have already been harmed. Outcome data can illuminate what went wrong, but it rarely provides early warning of emerging vulnerabilities.

This limitation has also been recognized in research on high-reliability organizations. High-reliability organization theory emerged from the study of high-hazard settings such as nuclear power and air traffic control, where safety depends not only on investigating failure but also on maintaining sensitivity to operations and detecting instability early [4]. Healthcare systems increasingly recognize the need for similar capabilities.

## Leading Indicators: Detecting System Strain

If serious safety events function as lagging indicators of safety performance, anticipatory patient safety systems require a complementary set of signals that reveal strain before harm occurs. These signals are often subtle. They rarely appear in formal safety dashboards and are frequently dismissed as routine operational friction. Yet within complex sociotechnical systems, small deviations from expected workflow frequently represent the earliest evidence that system conditions are becoming unstable.

Healthcare organizations encounter these signals every day. Clinicians request repeated clarifications during handoffs. Electronic alerts are dismissed in order to maintain workflow continuity. Documentation tasks accumulate during periods of high patient volume. Patients struggle to navigate discharge instructions or follow-up scheduling. None of these occurrences necessarily constitutes a patient safety event. Viewed individually, they appear minor. Viewed collectively, they reveal patterns of system strain that traditional outcome metrics cannot detect.

Human factors research has long demonstrated that performance degradation often emerges gradually as cognitive demand, environmental complexity, and workload increase [5]. When clinicians operate near the limits of attentional capacity, even small disruptions can cascade across tasks and decision points. The system continues to function, but its margin for safe performance narrows.

Leading indicators of fragility therefore focus on system conditions rather than discrete failures. Instead of measuring whether harm has occurred, they examine how reliably the system functions under multiple operational pressures. Measures of cognitive workload, communication reliability, workflow interruptions, and coordination delays offer insight into how the system behaves before failure becomes visible.

This perspective aligns with the broader shift in safety science from outcome-focused evaluation toward an understanding of everyday performance. Safety does not arise solely from the absence of error. It emerges from the ability of clinicians, teams, and organizations to adapt successfully to changing conditions [1].

Design-based inquiry methods introduced in the previous chapter provide a mechanism for detecting these signals. Contextual observation reveals where clinicians improvise to maintain workflow continuity. Journey mapping exposes friction across transitions in care. Service blueprinting clarifies dependencies between organizational layers that may not be visible in policy or protocol documentation. Together, these methods generate observational data that can be translated into indicators of emerging system strain.

Detecting these signals requires organizations to expand their definition of safety data. Incident reports and outcome metrics remain important, but they must be complemented by operational indicators that capture how work unfolds under real conditions. When aggregated and interpreted over time, these indicators provide a dynamic picture of system resilience. They reveal whether redesigned workflows reduce strain or whether hidden dependencies continue to accumulate risk. These signals become more actionable when organizations define the specific system conditions they want to observe and monitor over time.

Importantly, leading indicators are not intended to predict specific adverse events with precision. Complex adaptive systems rarely allow such deterministic forecasting. Their value lies instead in revealing patterns of instability early enough for organizations to intervene before failure becomes visible.

## Measuring System Conditions in Clinical Work

Capturing early signals of fragility requires expanding the types of data that healthcare organizations examine. Traditional safety dashboards emphasize outcomes such as infection rates, mortality, or serious safety events. While these indicators remain essential, they reveal little about how clinical systems behave under everyday operating conditions.

Anticipatory safety therefore requires attention to the system conditions that shape clinical work long before harm becomes visible.

### Workflow Reliability

Clinical care depends on complex sequences of interdependent tasks performed by multiple professionals across shifting clinical environments. Measurement of workflow reliability examines whether critical steps occur consistently and whether delays, workarounds, or repeated clarifications are becoming more common. Persistent variation in workflow execution often signals misalignment between formal process design and real operational conditions.

### Coordination Across Teams

Many safety failures arise at boundaries between professional groups or organizational units. Measurement of coordination patterns can reveal communication gaps during handoffs, delays in consultation responses, or ambiguity about responsibility during escalation events. Viewed individually, these coordination issues may appear operational rather than safety-related. Viewed collectively, they frequently precede serious breakdowns in care continuity.

### Cognitive Workload

Healthcare professionals routinely make high-stakes decisions under conditions of time pressure and information overload. Documentation burden, fragmented digital interfaces, and excessive alerting can increase cognitive workload and reduce situational awareness.

Research applying cognitive load theory to clinical environments demonstrates that increasing informational complexity can degrade decision performance even among experienced clinicians [5]. Measurement of documentation time, navigation complexity within electronic health records, and alert response patterns can therefore provide indirect signals of growing cognitive strain.

### Environmental Design and Workflow Friction

The physical environment also shapes how clinicians and patients interact with care systems. Equipment placement, visibility of monitoring displays, lighting, noise levels, and room configuration all influence how reliably clinicians can perform critical tasks. Human factors research has repeatedly demonstrated that design features of the work environment affect attention, coordination, and task completion reliability [6].

Together, these indicators provide a more dynamic picture of system stability. They reveal whether redesigned processes reduce operational strain or whether new vulnerabilities continue to emerge as conditions evolve.

## New Sources of Safety Insight

### Digital Exhaust and Behavioral Signals in Healthcare Systems

Modern healthcare systems generate enormous volumes of data through electronic health records, clinical monitoring devices, real-time location systems, scheduling platforms, and communication systems. Much of this information is produced as a by-product of routine activity rather than as intentional measurement. Researchers increasingly refer to these traces as digital exhaust, reflecting the behavioral signals embedded within everyday interactions with digital infrastructure.

Electronic health record systems, for example, capture detailed metadata about how clinicians interact with patient information. These log files record when charts are opened, how long clinicians spend reviewing laboratory results, how frequently alerts are overridden, and how documentation tasks are sequenced across a shift. When analyzed collectively, these data reveal patterns of workflow behavior that are rarely visible through traditional patient safety reporting mechanisms.

Emerging research using electronic health record audit logs demonstrates that metadata generated during routine clinical work can reveal patterns of workflow fragmentation, documentation burden, and alert interaction that may contribute to clinician cognitive workload and system reliability [7, 8]. High rates of alert overrides may indicate poorly calibrated decision support systems. Extended navigation time between critical data elements may signal interface complexity that disrupts clinical reasoning. Clusters of after-hours documentation activity may reflect workload patterns that increase cognitive fatigue. These behavioral signals allow organizations to observe how clinicians interact with the infrastructure of care itself.

## Emerging Sensing Technologies in Healthcare

Advances in sensing technologies are beginning to expand the range of behavioral signals available for patient safety monitoring. Environmental sensors, wearable devices, location-tracking systems, and computer vision tools can capture patterns of patient mobility, clinician movement through care environments, and delays in response to patient needs. Recent reviews suggest that these digital approaches are increasingly being explored in hospital and long-term care settings, although effectiveness and implementation remain variable across contexts [9].

For example, motion-sensing and computer vision systems can identify repeated attempts by a patient to exit the bed unassisted, changes in posture, or movement patterns associated with heightened fall risk. In one 2025 hospital evaluation, an AI-based vision system that monitored patients in real time was associated with a significantly lower fall incidence in monitored patients than in unmonitored patients [10]. While these technologies remain early in their adoption, they illustrate how advances in sensing and analytics may expand the observability of healthcare systems and support earlier intervention [9].

## Illustrative Example: Sensor-Based Monitoring to Reduce Patient Fall Risk

Falls remain one of the most common safety risks in hospitalized patients, particularly among older adults with mobility limitations or cognitive impairment. Traditional fall-prevention strategies rely heavily on retrospective review of fall incidents, environmental checklists, and bedside precautions such as bed alarms or mobility assistance protocols. While these interventions reduce risk, they typically activate only after patients attempt to mobilize independently or after a fall has already occurred.

Recent advances in sensing technologies are beginning to expand how healthcare organizations monitor patient mobility. Motion sensors, wearable devices, and computer vision systems can capture patterns of patient movement within hospital rooms. Rather than relying solely on incident reporting, these systems generate continuous behavioral data describing how patients interact with their environment.

Artificial intelligence techniques are increasingly being applied to analyze these movement patterns. Vision-based systems can evaluate posture changes, gait instability, and abrupt shifts in body position that may signal elevated fall risk. Machine learning models trained in mobility data are capable of recognizing patterns associated with falls and triggering alerts to caregivers when high-risk movement occurs [9, 10].

Although many of these technologies currently focus on detecting falls as they occur, their underlying capability lies in recognizing behavioral signals that precede loss of balance or unsafe mobility attempts. As sensing technologies and analytical models improve, these systems may allow healthcare organizations to intervene earlier by notifying staff, modifying environmental conditions, or adjusting care plans before a fall occurs.

This example illustrates how advances in sensing and artificial intelligence may expand the observability of patient behavior within healthcare environments. When integrated with clinical workflows and safety monitoring systems, such technologies may contribute to more anticipatory approaches to fall prevention.

## Measuring System Resilience

### Adaptive Capacity and System Resilience

Healthcare organizations frequently evaluate patient safety by examining whether processes function as intended under stable conditions. Yet real clinical environments rarely remain stable for long. Patient volume fluctuates, staffing changes, information systems slow or fail, and urgent clinical decisions compress time for communication and verification. In these conditions, the ability of teams to adapt safely becomes a critical determinant of patient outcomes.

Safety science increasingly describes this capability as adaptive capacity. Rather than focusing exclusively on preventing disruptions, adaptive capacity examines how systems maintain safe performance when disruptions occur. Teams redistribute workload, adjust communication patterns, and modify task sequencing in order to stabilize care delivery. These adjustments are not deviations from safety; they are often the mechanisms through which safety is preserved [1].

Measurement that captures adaptive capacity therefore focuses on how systems respond to pressure rather than only whether failure occurs. Indicators may include the reliability of escalation pathways, the time required for teams to regain coordination after interruptions, or the ability of clinical units to redistribute workload during periods of surge. When examined over time, these measures reveal whether redesign efforts strengthen the system's ability to operate safely under varying conditions.

This perspective expands the definition of patient safety measurement. Lagging indicators reveal when serious safety events have occurred. Leading indicators expose early signals of system strain. Measures of adaptive capacity reveal whether the organization can sustain safe performance when those pressures inevitably arise. The next question, then, is how organizations evaluate whether design-driven interventions actually strengthen these capacities over time.

## Evaluating Design-Driven Patient Safety Interventions

The design methods described in the previous chapter produce insight into how clinical systems actually function under real conditions. Measurement completes this process by determining whether those insights translate into improved system performance.

In this way, design thinking and measurement form a continuous learning cycle. Design inquiry identifies system vulnerabilities. Prototypes test potential redesigns. Measurement determines whether those changes stabilize system performance over time.

When sustained, this cycle transforms patient safety improvement from isolated interventions into ongoing system learning.

## Mixed-Method Evaluation in Safety Redesign

Traditional patient safety evaluation often relies heavily on outcome metrics. An intervention is implemented, and organizations observe whether occurrence rates decline. While these indicators remain important, they rarely capture the full effects of system redesign.

Human factors research has repeatedly demonstrated that system design strongly influences cognitive performance and decision-making behavior [5]. Changes to information architecture, workflow sequencing, or staffing configuration can alter attentional demand and coordination requirements in ways that may not be immediately visible through traditional outcome measures. Evaluating design-driven interventions therefore requires attention to how *clinicians* experience the system as well as how patients experience the outcomes of care.

Qualitative insight plays an important role in this process. Observational follow-up allows organizations to examine whether the redesigned workflow functions as intended in real clinical environments. Teams may observe how clinicians interact with new processes, whether communication pathways remain clear under pressure, and whether new workarounds begin to emerge.

Quantitative measures complement these observations by revealing how system performance changes over time. Metrics may include task completion time, escalation response intervals, documentation burden, or coordination delays between care teams. When interpreted alongside observational insight, these measures provide a more complete understanding of whether redesign efforts improve reliability or merely relocate complexity elsewhere in the system.

Design-driven evaluation also emphasizes iterative learning rather than single-point assessment. Early prototypes may produce partial improvements while revealing new sources of strain. Measurement allows teams to detect these signals quickly and adjust the intervention before broader implementation. This cycle reflects the broader principles of adaptive patient safety systems, in which interventions are continually refined as operational conditions evolve [1].

Importantly, evaluation should not be limited to isolated project teams. Insights generated through design-based investigation must eventually inform broader organizational learning. When redesign efforts reveal structural dependencies such as workload thresholds, coordination bottlenecks, or technology limitations, those insights provide valuable information for future system planning. In this way, evaluation becomes a means of strengthening institutional understanding of how safety emerges within complex healthcare systems.

## Case Example: Closed-Loop Medication Safety

Medication administration represents one of the more complex and risk-sensitive processes in healthcare delivery. Prescribing, verification, dispensing, and administration involve multiple professionals and information systems operating across different clinical environments. Traditional medication safety programs have relied heavily on retrospective reporting of medication errors, pharmacy review processes, and periodic chart audits. While these mechanisms remain important, they often identify problems only after an error has already occurred.

Closed-loop medication management systems are designed to reduce this gap by embedding verification directly into the medication workflow. These systems integrate electronic prescribing, pharmacy information systems, barcode medication administration, and patient identification technologies to ensure that each step in the medication process is electronically validated before the next step proceeds.

In a closed-loop system, medication orders are entered electronically through computerized provider order entry. Pharmacists verify the order and dispense the medication with a barcode linked to the specific patient and medication record. At the bedside, clinicians scan both the patient's identification band and the medication barcode before administration. The system then confirms that the correct medication, dose, route, and timing match the active medication order.

Beyond preventing individual errors, closed-loop systems generate continuous data about how medications move through the clinical environment. Barcode scanning compliance, override patterns, timing delays between medication ordering and administration, and discrepancies detected during verification all provide insight into workflow reliability. Recent studies of closed-loop and barcode-enabled systems support the value of these data both for improving medication safety and for identifying barriers, noncompliance, and mismatch patterns that may signal workflow strain [11].

Studies of barcode medication administration systems have demonstrated substantial reductions in administration errors when closed-loop verification is consistently implemented [6, 12]. At the same time, the digital trace data generated through these systems can reveal broader system conditions. For example, repeated scanning overrides may indicate workflow friction, poorly designed medication packaging, or staffing pressures that encourage clinicians to bypass safety steps. Monitoring these signals allows organizations to identify emerging vulnerabilities within medication workflows before they manifest as serious safety events.

Closed-loop medication safety illustrates how measurement can be embedded directly into clinical processes. Rather than functioning solely as retrospective surveillance, safety monitoring becomes part of the operational infrastructure of care delivery. When integrated with broader patient safety analytics, these systems allow healthcare organizations to observe medication workflows continuously and respond to emerging risks with earlier redesign or targeted intervention.

### Illustrative Example: Using Audit Log Data to Redesign Clinical Decision Support

Clinical decision support systems are widely used to reduce medication errors and improve adherence to clinical guidelines. However, poorly calibrated alerts can interrupt workflow, contribute to documentation burden, and add to clinician cognitive load. Recent studies continue to show that alert burden remains substantial and that many alerts are overridden, often because they are poorly targeted or insufficiently relevant to the clinical context [13].

Audit log data offers one way to make these patterns visible. By examining metadata on alert firings, override behavior, documentation activity, and EHR interaction patterns, organizations can identify where digital systems create friction in everyday work. Research on EHR use and documentation burden suggests that these patterns can illuminate workflow fragmentation and other usability problems that are not obvious from outcome metrics alone [7, 8].

Recent optimization efforts have shown that when organizations combine behavioral data with structured governance and redesign, they can reduce unnecessary alert volume and improve the proportion of alerts that clinicians act on [13]. In this way, audit log analysis becomes a design input for improving usability and patient safety.

## Measurement as Organizational Learning

Design-driven safety work often begins at the local level. A clinical team redesigns a workflow to reduce medication reconciliation errors. A new escalation pathway improves response time during patient deterioration. These improvements can produce measurable benefits within the department where they originate. Yet the broader safety impact depends on whether the learning extends beyond the immediate project environment.

Healthcare organizations frequently struggle at this stage. Improvement efforts succeed locally but remain isolated from institutional decision-making. Teams produce valuable insight about workflow fragility, workload thresholds, or coordination barriers, but those insights do not always influence governance structures, budgeting decisions, or system-wide standards. As a result, organizations may solve the same problem repeatedly in different departments rather than translating learning into structural improvement.

Complex systems require mechanisms that allow local discovery to inform institutional understanding. Sociotechnical research has emphasized that safety outcomes emerge from interactions among multiple organizational layers rather than from isolated components [14]. Workflow redesign in one clinical unit may reveal technology limitations that affect the entire organization. A successful prototype may demonstrate staffing conditions required for safe care delivery across multiple services. When these insights remain localized, the organization loses an opportunity to strengthen system-wide reliability.

Translation begins with making operational insight legible to leadership. Design artifacts such as journey maps or service blueprints help teams understand complex processes, but executive audiences require a different form of communication. Leaders need to understand what the findings imply about system behavior. Which dependencies proved unstable? At what workload threshold did reliability degrade? Which coordination points created recurring vulnerability? Framing the results in terms of system conditions allows leadership teams to interpret redesign efforts as indicators of broader structural patterns.

Governance forums play an important role in this translation process. Traditional safety oversight often concentrates on retrospective event review, regulatory reporting, and compliance monitoring. These activities remain necessary, but they primarily illuminate past failure. Integrating insight from design-driven investigation expands the conversation. Weak signals observed during workflow redesign, stress responses uncovered during simulation testing, and cognitive workload indicators identified during observation can provide early evidence of emerging system strain.

Learning health system models emphasize this continuous feedback between frontline experience and organizational decision making [15]. Information generated through daily clinical work becomes a source of institutional learning rather than remaining confined to individual projects. When redesign insights inform strategic planning, technology governance, and workforce decisions, the organization begins to operate as an adaptive system rather than a collection of independent improvement efforts.

Resource allocation provides the clearest indicator that learning has reached the institutional level. If redesign efforts consistently demonstrate that patient safety deteriorates beyond a specific workload threshold, staffing models become safety variables rather than purely operational metrics. If interface testing reveals that cognitive overload occurs within certain documentation structures, information architecture becomes a governance concern rather than a local usability issue. Human factors research has shown that interface design strongly influences cognitive performance and clinical decision making, reinforcing why these insights must inform system-level technology decisions [6].

Institutional memory is equally important. Many improvement efforts generate valuable findings that fade once the initial project concludes. Without mechanisms to preserve these lessons, organizations risk repeating the same experiments in different departments. Establishing repositories of tested assumptions, validated workflow changes, and documented system vulnerabilities allows knowledge to accumulate over time. Instead of episodic improvement, the organization builds a growing body of operational understanding that strengthens anticipatory safety capacity.

Safety science increasingly recognizes that healthcare organizations function as complex adaptive systems in which reliability depends on continuous learning rather than static control [3]. Translating local redesign insight into system-level knowledge is therefore not a secondary step in improvement work. It is the process through which individual interventions contribute to long-term organizational resilience.

## Sustaining Adaptive Patient Safety Systems

Measurement systems in healthcare are often designed for stability. Indicators are defined, dashboards are constructed, and performance is tracked over time. These structures are necessary for accountability and transparency, yet they can also create the impression that safety can be managed through fixed metrics alone. In complex clinical systems, reliability depends less on static measurement and more on the organization's ability to interpret signals and adapt accordingly.

Adaptive safety systems treat measurement as an ongoing process of inquiry rather than a final assessment of performance. Indicators are not only tools for confirming improvement but also instruments for detecting emerging strains. Small shifts in workflow timing, communication clarity, cognitive demand, or coordination reliability may signal changes in system behavior long before serious safety events occur. Monitoring these signals requires organizations to view data as part of a dynamic learning process rather than as a static record of past performance.

This perspective aligns with contemporary safety science, which emphasizes that resilience emerges from an organization's capacity to monitor, respond, learn, and anticipate within complex operational environments [1]. Measurement systems therefore function also as sensing mechanisms. They help organizations detect when conditions are drifting away from the assumptions that originally supported safe performance.

Sustaining this capability requires deliberate integration between measurement practices and the design methods described in the previous chapters. Observational insights gathered through contextual inquiry, journey mapping, and workflow analysis provide qualitative signals about system strain. Quantitative indicators such as response times, escalation frequency, workload measures, or documentation burden provide complementary evidence about how system conditions are evolving. When these sources of information are interpreted together, organizations gain a richer understanding of how safety emerges within everyday clinical work.

Equally important is the ability to revisit previously successful interventions. Healthcare environments do not remain static. Staffing models evolve, technology platforms change, and patient populations shift over time. An intervention that improves safety under one set of conditions may perform differently when those conditions change. Periodic reassessment allows organizations to confirm whether safety gains persist or whether redesign is required to maintain reliability.

Institutional leadership plays a central role in sustaining this learning cycle. Executive oversight of safety metrics often focuses on high-level outcomes such as event rates or regulatory indicators. While these measures remain essential, leaders who oversee adaptive safety systems also pay attention to operational signals generated through frontline design work. Observational findings, weak signals detected during workflow analysis, and insights generated through prototyping can reveal emerging risks that have not yet produced measurable harm. Incorporating these signals into governance conversations strengthens the organization's ability to respond before failures accumulate.

Over time, organizations that combine disciplined measurement with design-driven inquiry begin to develop a deeper understanding of their own operational patterns. They learn where coordination tends to break down, which technologies introduce cognitive strain, and which environmental conditions influence reliability. This accumulated knowledge allows leaders and clinicians to anticipate challenges more effectively and to redesign systems before those challenges manifest as patient harm.

Patient safety improvement has advanced in large part through careful analysis of failure. That work remains essential. The next stage depends on whether retrospective investigation can be supplemented by forms of learning that are more prospective, more continuous, and more attentive to how systems are behaving before serious harm becomes visible. Measurement, when it is integrated with observation and redesign, is one of the means by which that becomes possible.

The aim is not to eliminate uncertainty from complex healthcare environments. That would be neither realistic nor desirable in adaptive systems that must respond to diverse patient needs and changing conditions. The more practical task is to ensure that organizations remain attentive to how their systems behave under real pressures and are prepared to redesign those systems as those pressures evolve.

In that sense, measurement becomes more than a tool for evaluating improvement after the fact. It becomes part of an ongoing practice of stewardship. Through observation, analysis, and redesign carried out over time, healthcare organizations can move toward a form of patient safety that is more anticipatory, more adaptive, and more closely grounded in the realities of clinical work.

## References


1. Hollnagel E. Safety-I and Safety-II: the past and future of safety management. Farnham: Ashgate Publishing; 2014.
2. Lipsitz LA. Understanding health care as a complex system: the foundation for unintended consequences. JAMA. 2012;308(3):243–4. https://doi.org/10.1001/jama.2012.7551.
3. Young RA, Xiao Y, Fulda KG. Safety-I versus Safety-II: a mixed-methods study revealing the imbalance of approaches in primary care medication safety. J Patient Saf. 2025;21(Suppl 1):S81–8. https://doi.org/10.1097/PTS.0000000000001259.
4. Dwyer J, Staines A, McMahon M. Scoping review of peer-reviewed empirical studies on implementing high reliability organisation theory. Saf Sci. 2023;166:106239.
5. Young JQ, Van Merriënboer J, Durning S, Ten Cate O. Cognitive load theory: implications for medical education. Med Educ. 2014;48(3):225–34. https://doi.org/10.1111/medu.12373.
6. Carayon P, Wooldridge A, Hoonakker P, Hundt AS, Kelly MM. SEIPS 3.0: human-centered design of the patient journey for patient safety. Appl Ergon. 2020;84:103033. https://doi.org/10.1016/j.apergo.2019.103033.
7. Asgari E, Kaur J, Nuredini G, Balloch J, Taylor AM, Sebire N, Robinson R, Peters C, Sridharan S, Pimenta D. Impact of electronic health record use on cognitive load and burnout among clinicians: narrative review. JMIR Med Inform. 2024;12:e55499. https://doi.org/10.2196/55499.
8. Moy AJ, Schwartz JM, Chen R, Sadri S, Lucas E, Cato KD, et al. Measurement of clinician EHR use with audit logs: a scoping review. J Am Med Inform Assoc. 2023;30(3):564–75. https://doi.org/10.1093/jamia/ocac214.

9. Lee A, Lee H, Lee SH. Digital healthcare approaches for fall detection and prediction in older adults: a systematic review of evidence from hospital and long-term care settings. Medicina (Kaunas). 2025;61(11):1926. https://doi.org/10.3390/medicina61111926.
10. Gervasi C, Perego E, Galli F, Torri V, Castoldi M, Bombardieri E. Prevention of falls in hospitalized patients: evaluation of the effectiveness of a monitoring system (Verso Vision) developed with artificial intelligence. Front Digit Health. 2025;7:1548209. https://doi.org/10.3389/fdgth.2025.1548209.
11. Yin X, Song H, Lu J, Yang J, Wang R, Lin Z, Jiang S, Yuan H, Wang X, Xu D, Gao C, Zhou Y, Xu J, Chen C, Gu C, Diao Q, Li F, Gu Z. Effect of a closed-loop medication order executive system on safe medication administration at a tertiary hospital: a quasi-experimental study. Ther Adv Drug Saf. 2024;15:20420986241288421. https://doi.org/10.1177/20420986241288421.
12. Poon EG, Keohane CA, Yoon CS, et al. Effect of barcode technology on the safety of medication administration. N Engl J Med. 2010;362:1698–707. https://doi.org/10.1056/NEJMsa0907115.
13. Ng HJH, Kansal A, Abdul Naseer JF, Hing WC, Goh CJM, Poh H, D'Souza JLA, Lim EL, Tan G. Optimizing Best Practice Advisory alerts in electronic medical records with a multi-pronged strategy at a tertiary care hospital in Singapore. JAMIA Open. 2023;6(3):ooad056. https://doi.org/10.1093/jamiaopen/ooad056.
14. Papoutsi C, Reed JE, Marston C, Lewis R, Majeed A, Bell D. Patient safety and the sociotechnical perspective: past, present, and future. BMJ Qual Saf. 2020;29(5):419–25. https://doi.org/10.1136/bmjqs-2019-009485.
15. Platt JE, Raj M, Wienroth M, McGowan ML. Embedding a learning health system approach within healthcare organizations. Learn Health Syst. 2022;6(2):e10288. https://doi.org/10.1002/lrh2.10288.

# Building a Culture of Anticipation

# 10

## From Improvement Projects to Institutional Capability

Patient safety science increasingly recognizes that improving safety requires more than analyzing events after harm has occurred [1]. Healthcare delivery unfolds within complex systems shaped by evolving technologies, interdisciplinary teamwork, operational pressures, and changing patient needs [2]. In such environments, safety depends on identifying failure and on understanding how clinical systems behave under everyday conditions [3]. The central challenge is therefore not simply improving individual processes but developing the organizational capability to continually examine and redesign the systems through which care is delivered using structured methods for observing and understanding real-world clinical work.

Methods such as contextual observation, journey mapping, service blueprinting, assumption testing, and structured validation provide practical ways to investigate how work actually unfolds within clinical environments [4]. Measurement systems then allow teams to determine whether redesign efforts improve reliability and reduce system strain [5]. Together, these approaches enable healthcare organizations to move beyond retrospective investigation toward a more anticipatory model of patient safety stewardship.



K. Rasmussen, *Rethinking Patient Safety*,
https://doi.org/10.1007/978-3-032-26054-3_10

Yet generating insight through redesign does not automatically produce system-wide change. A clinical team may identify coordination barriers that delay escalation of care. A unit may redesign a workflow that reduces cognitive burden during medication reconciliation. A prototype may demonstrate how interface changes improve clinician awareness of patient deterioration. These discoveries can meaningfully improve safety within the settings where they originate. However, the institutional structures that shape safety across the organization often remain unchanged.

Research in healthcare quality improvement has consistently shown that locally successful interventions often struggle to spread or sustain when the organizational conditions required for adoption are not addressed, including leadership alignment, resource availability, and integration with existing workflows [1, 6–8]. The result is a familiar pattern in healthcare improvement: valuable insight emerges within individual projects while the larger system continues to operate according to the same assumptions that produced the original vulnerability.

Addressing this challenge requires shifting the focus of patient safety work from isolated initiatives to institutional capability. Anticipatory safety depends on organizations that can detect early signals of system strain, interpret those signals through disciplined inquiry, and respond through deliberate redesign of care processes and infrastructure. In this sense, anticipatory patient safety is best understood as an organizational capability rather than a discrete safety program. The ability to examine system behavior, interpret emerging signals, and redesign care processes must become embedded within how the organization operates.

Healthcare systems that demonstrate this capacity tend to develop three reinforcing organizational capabilities. Governance structures must prioritize early detection of system fragility rather than relying solely on retrospective event analysis [9]. The workforce must possess the skills necessary to observe work as it occurs, interpret weak signals, and participate in structured redesign of clinical systems. Finally, organizations must establish learning mechanisms that translate operational insight into institutional decision-making so that discoveries made in one setting inform system-level change [10, 11].

These capabilities rarely emerge spontaneously. Healthcare institutions have historically built safety programs around mechanisms designed to respond to harm after it occurs. Incident reporting systems, event investigations, and regulatory oversight have strengthened accountability and transparency across the field, but they primarily illuminate failures that have already occurred [12, 13]. Anticipatory safety expands this framework by directing attention toward the system conditions that precede harm and by strengthening the organizational capacity to respond before vulnerabilities escalate into patient injury [3].

Building this capacity requires changes in how healthcare organizations lead, train, and learn. Leadership structures must shift from event-centered oversight toward continuous examination of system behavior. Clinicians and operational leaders must develop the skills necessary to investigate complex sociotechnical environments and participate in redesign efforts. Institutional learning mechanisms must ensure that insights generated through local redesign efforts inform policy, resource allocation, and system-wide standards. When these elements align, patient safety evolves from a reactive function focused on investigation to an organizational capability centered on anticipation.

## Governance for Anticipatory Patient Safety

Patient safety governance has traditionally focused on the investigation of adverse outcomes. Safety committees review incident reports, regulatory bodies establish reporting requirements, and organizational leaders examine event summaries to determine whether corrective action is required. These mechanisms have strengthened accountability and improved the transparency of safety oversight across healthcare systems [3, 13]. They ensure that serious safety events receive formal investigation and that organizations remain attentive to patterns of harm.

However, governance structures designed primarily around retrospective event analysis face inherent limitations when applied to complex clinical systems. By the time an adverse outcome becomes visible through reporting systems, the conditions that enabled it have often been developing for extended periods. Workflow misalignment, cognitive overload, coordination failures, and technology friction may accumulate gradually before eventually manifesting as patient harm [2, 12]. Event review can illuminate these contributing factors, but it rarely provides early visibility into their emergence.

Anticipatory safety governance therefore expands the scope of oversight beyond the investigation of individual events. Leadership attention must also focus on the conditions under which care is delivered and the signals that suggest increasing system strain. These signals may appear as recurring workarounds, repeated clarification during handoffs, rising documentation burden, technology navigation delays, or staffing patterns that push clinicians toward sustained cognitive overload. Individually, such signals may appear operational rather than safety-related. When examined collectively, they provide insight into how system conditions are evolving.

This changes the questions that leaders ask when examining safety performance. Instead of focusing exclusively on whether an adverse event has occurred, governance structures must also consider where fragility may be accumulating within the system. This requires integrating observational insight, operational data, and workforce experience into safety discussions that have historically relied primarily on event reporting and compliance indicators. When governance forums examine system conditions in addition to outcomes, organizations become better positioned to detect emerging risk before harm occurs.

Leadership structures also influence how redesign insights are translated into organizational action. Frontline teams may identify workflow dependencies, technology limitations, or staffing constraints that affect safety performance. Without governance mechanisms capable of interpreting and acting on those insights, redesign efforts remain localized. When leadership bodies incorporate operational insight into strategic decision-making, discoveries made in one clinical setting can inform policy, resource allocation, and system design across the organization [9, 13].

Developing governance structures that support anticipatory safety therefore represents a central step in building institutional capability. Oversight must extend beyond the investigation of failure to include continuous attention to how systems behave under real conditions. When leaders examine system performance through this broader lens, patient safety becomes less dependent on reacting to harm and more focused on identifying and redesigning the conditions that allow harm to occur.

## Developing Design Capability in Healthcare Teams

Governance structures can prioritize anticipatory safety, but leadership attention alone cannot sustain it. The ability to detect system fragility and redesign clinical processes ultimately depends on the people who work within the system every day. Clinicians, operational leaders, and support staff experience the practical realities of care delivery in ways that formal policy or performance dashboards cannot fully capture. When those individuals possess the skills necessary to examine system behavior and participate in redesign, organizations gain a powerful source of operational insight.

Healthcare professionals, however, are not typically trained in systems investigation methods as part of standard clinical or operational education. Clinical education focuses appropriately on diagnosis, treatment, and patient care. Administrative training usually emphasizes operational efficiency and regulatory compliance. These competencies are essential, yet they do not necessarily equip teams to examine how workflows evolve, how technologies influence cognition, or how coordination patterns shift across complex care environments [14]. As a result, organizations frequently rely on a small number of specialists to conduct improvement work while the broader workforce remains primarily engaged in day-to-day operations.

Anticipatory safety requires expanding this capability across the organization. Clinicians and operational leaders must develop the ability to observe work as it unfolds, interpret patterns of adaptation and strain, and participate in structured redesign of care processes. The methods described earlier in this book provide one pathway for developing those skills. Contextual observation reveals how clinicians adapt to real conditions. Journey mapping highlights how patients and staff experience care transitions. Service blueprinting clarifies how workflows, technologies, and organizational structures interact. When used with discipline, these approaches enable teams to examine system performance in ways that traditional audit or compliance mechanisms cannot capture [4, 14].

Importantly, developing design capability does not require transforming clinicians into professional designers. Instead, it involves equipping healthcare teams with investigative and analytical skills that complement their clinical expertise. Physicians, nurses, pharmacists, and allied health professionals already possess a deep understanding of patient care processes. When these professionals are trained to examine systems with the same rigor they apply to clinical reasoning, they can identify subtle vulnerabilities that may not be visible to external analysts or improvement specialists.

Some healthcare organizations have created structures that support this type of interdisciplinary investigation. Innovation centers, experience design programs, and clinical redesign laboratories provide environments where clinicians collaborate with designers, engineers, and human factors specialists to examine care processes and prototype potential improvements [14]. More importantly, these structures demonstrate that redesign capability can become embedded within healthcare organizations rather than remaining confined to isolated improvement projects.

Workforce capability also influences how organizations respond to emerging safety signals. When clinicians are encouraged and equipped to surface observations about workflow friction, cognitive overload, or coordination barriers, those insights can inform redesign before harm occurs. Teams are more likely to engage in this type of learning behavior when the climate supports interpersonal candor and shared inquiry rather than punishment or silence [15]. Without this capability, early signals of system strain may be dismissed as routine operational challenges rather than recognized as indicators of deeper structural misalignment.

Developing design capability therefore represents a critical step in building a culture of anticipation. Governance structures may create the conditions for anticipatory safety, but the workforce provides the observational insight and redesign capacity that make those structures effective. When clinicians, operational leaders, and technical specialists collaborate to examine system behavior, organizations gain the ability to continuously refine how care is delivered in response to evolving conditions.

## Learning Systems for Continuous Patient Safety Adaptation

Governance structures can direct leadership attention toward emerging system conditions, and workforce capability allows clinicians and operational teams to investigate how care is actually delivered. Yet anticipatory patient safety cannot be sustained without mechanisms that convert operational insight into organizational learning. Discoveries made through observation, redesign, and validation must influence how the organization interprets risk, allocates resources, and updates the structures that guide care delivery.

Healthcare organizations frequently generate valuable insight through improvement work, but that insight does not always persist beyond the original project. A redesign effort may reveal that certain staffing patterns increase coordination failures during high patient volume. A workflow analysis may demonstrate that particular documentation structures increase cognitive load during critical decision points. These findings can produce immediate local improvements, yet they may fade once the project concludes unless mechanisms exist to preserve and interpret the knowledge that has been generated.

Learning systems address this challenge by ensuring that operational insight becomes part of institutional memory. Observations gathered through redesign initiatives can be documented, evaluated, and incorporated into broader decision-making processes. Measurement systems allow organizations to monitor how system conditions evolve over time, while governance forums provide opportunities to interpret these signals and determine whether redesign is necessary. When these processes function together, improvement work becomes cumulative rather than episodic.

In this way, safety improvement begins to resemble a learning cycle rather than a sequence of isolated projects. Observations from clinical work generate insight, insight informs redesign, and redesigned systems are then evaluated under real conditions. This type of learning infrastructure reflects principles associated with learning health systems, in which knowledge generated during routine operations continuously informs system redesign and policy development [10, 11]. It is also consistent with Safety-II literature that emphasizes learning from everyday work, including the adaptations that help clinical systems succeed under variable conditions [16].

Institutional learning also reduces the likelihood that organizations repeatedly encounter the same vulnerabilities. Without mechanisms for preserving insight, similar workflow problems may be investigated independently across multiple departments, each time requiring new analysis and redesign. By contrast, when knowledge from redesign initiatives is systematically documented and shared, organizations can recognize recurring structural patterns and address them at the system level. Recent work on organizational learning from failure reinforces that learning is shaped not only by the event itself but also by contextual factors such as workload, communication, and organizational conditions [17].

The development of learning infrastructure therefore strengthens anticipatory safety in two ways. First, it ensures that insights generated through frontline redesign efforts influence leadership decision-making and organizational policy. Second, it allows knowledge to accumulate across improvement initiatives, creating a growing body of understanding about how the system behaves under different conditions. Over time, this accumulation of insight enables organizations to anticipate emerging risks more effectively and redesign systems before those risks manifest as harm.

## Structural Barriers to Anticipatory Patient Safety

While the capabilities described in this chapter provide a foundation for anticipatory patient safety, implementing them within healthcare organizations is not straightforward. Clinical systems operate under structural constraints and intense operational pressure, both of which make proactive investigation and redesign difficult to sustain. Staffing shortages, fluctuating patient demand, and administrative requirements often consume the attention of leaders and frontline teams. Under such conditions, improvement work can be perceived as an additional responsibility rather than as an integral component of care delivery [7, 8].

Regulatory environments can also influence how safety is managed. Many oversight structures emphasize compliance with reporting requirements and corrective action following adverse events. These mechanisms play an important role in accountability, yet they may inadvertently reinforce a reactive orientation toward safety management [12, 13]. Organizations may focus significant effort on documenting incidents and implementing corrective policies while dedicating less attention to examining the conditions that give rise to vulnerability within everyday clinical work.

Digital infrastructure presents another challenge. Modern healthcare delivery depends on complex information systems that influence clinical decision-making, communication, and documentation. These technologies often evolve incrementally through vendor updates, regulatory requirements, and internal customization. As a result, digital workflows may become fragmented over time, introducing navigation complexity, alert burden, and documentation friction. Addressing these issues frequently requires coordination across technical, operational, and clinical leadership. Without governance structures capable of managing these interdependencies, redesign efforts may remain limited to local adjustments rather than producing broader improvements in system performance [14].

Workforce fatigue represents an additional barrier. Clinicians and support staff routinely operate under high cognitive and emotional demands. When organizations rely heavily on professional vigilance to maintain safe performance, opportunities for proactive investigation and redesign may be limited. Recent synthesis work identifies alarm fatigue as a significant risk to both patient safety and the well-being of healthcare professionals, illustrating how information overload can undermine both safe performance and improvement capacity [18]. Anticipatory safety depends on creating conditions in which clinicians can reflect on how systems function, in addition to whether tasks are completed. Providing time, support, and institutional encouragement for this type of inquiry is essential if redesign capability is to become embedded within daily operations.

Organizational inertia can further complicate change. Healthcare institutions often develop deeply established routines that shape how decisions are made and how work is organized. Policies, reporting structures, and technology platforms may reinforce these routines over time. While such stability can support reliability, it can also make redesign efforts difficult to implement when they challenge existing assumptions about how care should be delivered. Organizational readiness for change also matters. Recent review evidence shows that healthcare organizations vary considerably in how prepared their members feel to implement change in routine work, and that this variation can influence whether change efforts gain traction or stall [19].

Recognizing these barriers does not diminish the importance of anticipatory safety. Instead, it clarifies the conditions under which organizational capability must develop. Governance structures must create space for inquiry despite operational pressures. Workforce development must equip clinicians to interpret system behavior within complex environments. Learning mechanisms must ensure that insights generated through redesign efforts influence broader institutional decision-making. When these elements align, organizations can gradually shift from responding to harm after it occurs toward identifying and addressing the conditions that allow harm to emerge.

## Conclusion

Building a culture of anticipation requires more than the introduction of new methods. It requires healthcare organizations that can observe their own systems with some regularity, interpret what they are seeing with sufficient discipline, and respond before harm becomes the first unmistakable signal that something is wrong. That is a more demanding standard than retrospective review, not because retrospective work is unimportant, but because anticipation asks institutions to act while fragility is still emerging and while the evidence may be less dramatic than an adverse event.

The barriers to this work are real. Operational pressure narrows attention. Regulatory expectations continue to privilege visible events. Technology introduces new forms of complexity even as it promises greater visibility. Fatigue and overload reduce the space available for reflection. For those reasons, a culture of anticipation does not emerge quickly or evenly. It develops through repeated decisions about what the organization treats as worthy of attention and what kinds of signals it is prepared to act on.

What distinguishes anticipatory organizations is not that they prevent every form of failure. It is that they become better able to notice strain while the system is still holding, better able to learn from ordinary work rather than extraordinary breakdown alone, and more willing to redesign care processes before those processes fail publicly. That marks a substantial shift in how patient safety is understood. It is also, increasingly, a necessary one.

## References

1. Dixon-Woods M, McNicol S, Martin G. Ten challenges in improving quality in healthcare: lessons from the Health Foundation's programme evaluations and relevant literature. BMJ Qual Saf. 2012;21(10):876–84. https://doi.org/10.1136/bmjqs-2011-000760.
2. Lipsitz LA. Understanding health care as a complex system: the foundation for unintended consequences. JAMA. 2012;308(3):243–4. https://doi.org/10.1001/jama.2012.7551.

3. Hollnagel E. Safety-I and safety-II: the past and future of safety management. Farnham: Ashgate Publishing; 2014.
4. Carayon P, Wooldridge A, Hoonakker P, Hundt AS, Kelly MM. SEIPS 3.0: human-centered design of the patient journey for patient safety. Appl Ergon. 2020;84:103033. https://doi.org/10.1016/j.apergo.2019.103033.
5. Pronovost PJ, Holzmueller CG, Needham DM, Sexton JB, Miller M, Berenholtz S, et al. How will we know patients are safer? An organization-wide approach to measuring and improving safety. Crit Care Med. 2006;34(7):1988–95. https://doi.org/10.1097/01.CCM.0000226412.12612.B6.
6. Coles E, Anderson J, Maxwell M, Harris F, Gray NM, Milner G, et al. The influence of contextual factors on healthcare quality improvement initiatives: a realist review. Syst Rev. 2020;9(1):94. https://doi.org/10.1186/s13643-020-01344-3.
7. Lennox L, Maher L, Reed J. Navigating the sustainability landscape: a systematic review of sustainability approaches in healthcare. Implement Sci. 2018;13(1):27. https://doi.org/10.1186/s13012-017-0707-4.
8. Moon SEJ, Hogden A, Eljiz K. Sustaining improvement of hospital-wide initiative for patient safety and quality: a systematic scoping review. BMJ Open Qual. 2022;11(4):e002057. https://doi.org/10.1136/bmjoq-2022-002057.
9. Murray JS, Baghdadi A, Dannenberg W, Crews P, DeZellar WN. The role of high reliability organization foundational practices in building a culture of safety. Fed Pract. 2024;41(7):214–21. https://doi.org/10.12788/fp.0486.
10. Platt JE, Raj M, Wienroth M, McGowan ML. Embedding a learning health system approach within healthcare organizations. Learn Health Syst. 2022;6(2):e10288. https://doi.org/10.1002/lrh2.10288.
11. Kilbourne AM, Borsky AE, O'Brien RW, et al. The foundational science of learning health systems. Health Serv Res. 2024;59(6):e14374. https://doi.org/10.1111/1475-6773.14374.
12. Macrae C. The problem with incident reporting. BMJ Qual Saf. 2016;25(2):71–5. https://doi.org/10.1136/bmjqs-2015-004732.
13. World Health Organization. Global patient safety report 2024. Geneva: World Health Organization; 2024.
14. Awad S, Begg R, Loveday T, Baysari MT. Using human centred design and human factors to support a rapid health information technology patient safety response. BMC Health Serv Res. 2025;25(1):1143. https://doi.org/10.1186/s12913-025-13293-5.
15. Edmondson A. Psychological safety and learning behavior in work teams. Adm Sci Q. 1999;44(2):350–83. https://doi.org/10.2307/2666999.
16. Birkeli G, Lindahl AK, Hammersoen AM, Deilkas ECT, Ballangrud R. Strategies and tools to learn from work that goes well within healthcare patient safety practices: a mixed methods systematic review. BMC

Health Serv Res. 2025;25(1):538. https://doi.org/10.1186/s12913-025-12680-2.
17. Horck S. Interactions between the context of a health-care organisation and failure: the situational impact of failure on organisational learning. Leadersh Health Serv. 2024;37(4):595–610. https://doi.org/10.1108/LHS-04-2024-0036.
18. Michels EAM, Gilbert S, et al. Alarm fatigue in healthcare: a scoping review of definitions, influencing factors, and mitigation strategies. BMC Nurs. 2025;24(1):664. https://doi.org/10.1186/s12912-025-03369-2.
19. Caci L, Aubin K, Marcoux V, et al. Organizational readiness for change: a systematic review of the healthcare literature. Implement Res Pract. 2025;6:26334895251334536. https://doi.org/10.1177/26334895251334536.

# Patient Safety Reimagined: Designing the Future of Healthcare

# 11

## Introduction

Healthcare systems around the world are entering a period of unprecedented complexity. Advances in digital technologies, expanding clinical knowledge, demographic shifts, and evolving models of care are transforming how healthcare is delivered. These developments hold tremendous promise for improving outcomes and expanding access to care. At the same time, they introduce new forms of system interdependence, information overload, and operational strain. Within such environments, approaches to patient safety that rely primarily on investigating adverse events after harm occurs are increasingly insufficient. As healthcare systems grow more complex, the ability to anticipate early signals of risk becomes as important as the ability to respond to failures that have already occurred.

The modern patient safety movement has made substantial progress in identifying the causes of preventable harm. Landmark reports such as *To Err Is Human* demonstrated that adverse events frequently arise not from isolated mistakes but from failures within complex systems of care delivery [1]. Subsequent research in safety science reinforced this understanding by showing that human error often reflects interactions between individuals, technologies, organizational structures, and environmental conditions rather than the shortcomings of any single actor [2]. These insights



K. Rasmussen, *Rethinking Patient Safety*,
https://doi.org/10.1007/978-3-032-26054-3_11

helped shift the focus of patient safety from individual blame toward system design.

Understanding failure after harm occurs, however, represents only one dimension of safety improvement. Healthcare organizations frequently investigate adverse events through root cause analysis and incident reporting systems. These mechanisms remain essential for transparency and accountability, yet they primarily illuminate failures that have already occurred. Safety researchers increasingly argue that healthcare must also develop the capacity to understand how work unfolds during everyday clinical practice and how risks emerge before harm becomes visible [3, 4].

This book argues that anticipatory patient safety does not emerge from a single intervention or program. Instead, it develops when healthcare organizations gain the ability to observe care systems, question underlying assumptions, and redesign processes in response to what they learn. The investigative methods explored throughout this book, including contextual observation, journey mapping, service blueprinting, assumption testing, and structured validation, provide practical tools for examining how care actually unfolds in real clinical environments. When these methods are combined with governance structures, workforce capability, and learning systems that support continuous redesign, patient safety begins to shift from a reactive activity toward an organizational capability grounded in anticipation.

Research on resilient healthcare emphasizes that safety depends not only on preventing failure but also on understanding how systems adapt under changing conditions [4, 5]. Global patient safety initiatives similarly emphasize the need for proactive approaches that identify risk earlier within care processes rather than relying solely on retrospective investigation [6]. As healthcare systems continue to evolve, organizations that cultivate the ability to observe, interpret, and redesign care environments will be better positioned to maintain safe performance as complexity increases.

## From Reactive Safety to System Design

Throughout this book, patient safety has been examined through investigative methods designed to help healthcare teams understand how care systems actually function. Techniques such as contextual observation, journey mapping, service blueprinting, assumption testing, and structured validation offer practical ways to examine complex care environments. Each method reveals different aspects of how technologies, workflows, communication structures, and human behavior interact within clinical settings.

Taken together, these approaches demonstrate a broader shift in how patient safety can be understood. Rather than focusing exclusively on the analysis of adverse events after harm occurs, these methods allow organizations to observe how care unfolds during everyday practice and identify risks before they result in harm. In this sense, the investigative methods discussed throughout the book represent not simply tools for improvement but a foundation for designing safer healthcare systems.

For decades, the patient safety movement has advanced through careful examination of harm. Event investigations, root cause analysis, and incident reporting systems have helped healthcare organizations understand how breakdowns occur within clinical environments. These approaches have strengthened accountability and revealed important patterns in communication failure, workflow design, and technology interaction. They have also established patient safety as a central priority within healthcare governance. Yet the systems through which care is delivered have rarely been designed with patient safety as their primary organizing principle.

This observation demonstrates a broader principle within safety science. Systems that evolve gradually can accumulate hidden weaknesses even when individual components function as intended. Human factors research demonstrates that interactions among tasks, technologies, organizational policies, and environmental conditions often determine whether safe performance is possible within complex work systems [7]. When these interactions are not intentionally designed, clinicians must rely on experience and adaptation to maintain safe performance under challenging conditions.

Traditional approaches to patient safety often respond to harm after it occurs. When an adverse event becomes visible, organizations investigate the incident, identify contributing factors, and implement corrective actions. This process has produced meaningful improvements in many areas of care delivery. Medication reconciliation processes, surgical safety checklists, and infection prevention protocols all emerged from careful investigation of previous failures.

However, reactive safety approaches also have limitations. Because they focus on visible failures, they may overlook early signals that indicate increasing system strain. Workflow misalignment, cognitive overload, communication delays, and technology friction often develop gradually before manifesting as adverse outcomes. By the time an event becomes visible through reporting systems, the conditions that enabled it may have been present for extended periods.

Safety researchers have increasingly emphasized the importance of understanding how systems function during everyday clinical work rather than examining failure alone [3, 4]. This perspective reflects the broader shift from Safety I, which focuses on preventing adverse outcomes, toward Safety-II, which seeks to understand how complex systems sustain safe performance despite variability and uncertainty [3]. Examining everyday clinical work allows organizations to detect early signals of risk and redesign care processes before harm occurs.

The chapters in this book have explored investigative methods that enable healthcare teams to examine system performance more directly. Contextual observation reveals how clinicians adapt to real conditions. Journey mapping highlights how patients and staff experience transitions across care environments. Service blueprinting clarifies how workflows, technologies, and organizational structures interact. Structured validation methods allow teams to test redesign ideas before implementing large-scale change.

These approaches demonstrate a shift toward intentionally designing care systems rather than allowing them to evolve without deliberate examination. Measurement frameworks allow organizations to evaluate whether redesign efforts improve reliability and reduce system strain. Governance structures, workforce capability, and institutional learning mechanisms ensure that insights generated through local redesign efforts influence policy and system design across the organization. When these elements align, anticipatory patient safety becomes less dependent on responding to harm after it occurs and more focused on shaping the conditions that allow safe care to emerge.

## Designing Healthcare for Anticipation

If healthcare systems were designed with anticipatory safety as a central organizing principle, their structure would differ substantially from the environments that characterize much of contemporary clinical care. Rather than relying primarily on retrospective investigation to identify vulnerabilities, organizations would develop the capacity to examine system behavior continuously and adjust structures before fragility accumulates.

A defining characteristic of anticipatory systems is the routine examination of work as it unfolds under real conditions. Clinical processes cannot be understood solely through policy documents, workflow diagrams, or performance dashboards. These representations describe how work is intended to occur, but they commonly fail to capture the adaptations that clinicians make when navigating complex and unpredictable environments.

Observational methods allow healthcare teams to examine how technologies, staffing models, and operational pressures interact during everyday clinical work. Contextual observation, shadowing, and journey mapping provide insight into the subtle adjustments clinicians make to maintain safe performance in the face of time pressure, information gaps, and coordination challenges. Such observations frequently reveal patterns that remain invisible within traditional performance metrics.

Safety science research consistently demonstrates that frontline professionals often compensate for system weaknesses through informal adaptations that preserve safe care delivery [4,

5]. These adaptations are rarely documented in formal policies, yet they represent an essential component of system resilience. When organizations investigate how these adaptations occur, they gain insight into areas where system design may be misaligned with the realities of clinical work.

## Designing Through Iteration and Testing

Anticipatory systems approach change differently. Interventions are not implemented solely through policy directives or procedural updates. Instead, new workflows, technologies, and care models undergo structured testing before large-scale deployment.

Simulation environments, prototype testing, and iterative validation allow organizations to evaluate how proposed changes interact with real clinical conditions. These approaches reflect principles commonly used in engineering and design disciplines, where systems are tested under variable conditions before being implemented in high-risk environments. In healthcare, such testing can reveal unintended consequences that might otherwise remain undetected until after widespread implementation.

## Integrating Human Factors into System Design

Another defining feature of anticipatory healthcare systems is the integration of human factors expertise into routine organizational decision-making. Clinical environments place substantial cognitive demands on healthcare professionals. Documentation systems, alert mechanisms, communication channels, and workflow structures all influence how clinicians perceive information and make decisions.

Human factors research demonstrates that poorly designed systems can increase cognitive workload, fragment attention, and contribute to error even when clinicians are highly skilled and motivated [7]. Anticipatory organizations therefore evaluate how technologies and workflows interact with human cognition before implementing large-scale change. Emerging patient safety work in health information technology similarly reinforces the importance of human-centered design and human factors approaches when organizations introduce new digital tools into clinical environments [8].

This perspective encourages healthcare leaders to examine how design decisions influence the cognitive environment of clinical work. Questions such as how information is displayed, how alerts are prioritized, and how documentation requirements shape workflow can significantly influence clinical decision-making. When these elements are designed with an understanding of human cognitive limits, systems are better able to support safe performance under pressure.

## Learning from Patient and Family Experience

Anticipatory healthcare systems also treat patient and family experience as an important source of safety insight. Patients and caregivers frequently observe discontinuities in care that remain invisible to clinicians or administrators. Confusing instructions, repeated explanations, inconsistent information, and unclear coordination across care settings may signal underlying fragmentation within the care system.

Examining patient journeys across care environments allows organizations to identify these discontinuities and explore their underlying causes. Journey mapping techniques can reveal points where communication breaks down, where information must be repeated, or where responsibilities between care teams remain unclear.

When organizations systematically incorporate patient and family experience into redesign efforts, they gain a broader understanding of how care systems function across settings and over time. This perspective complements clinical observations by revealing system behaviors that emerge outside the boundaries of individual departments or encounters.

## Patient Safety in the Age of Intelligent Systems

Emerging technologies are often described as transformative forces within healthcare. Artificial intelligence, predictive analytics, advanced simulation environments, and digitally integrated monitoring systems are increasingly embedded within clinical practice. These tools have the potential to reshape how healthcare organizations detect and respond to emerging patient safety risks. However, technology alone does not produce safer systems. Its impact depends on how it is integrated into the broader design of clinical environments.

In anticipatory healthcare systems, technology becomes a mechanism for strengthening visibility into system behavior rather than merely accelerating clinical processes. Predictive analytics, for example, can identify patterns within operational and clinical data that signal emerging strain within care systems. Rising patient acuity, delayed response times, increasing documentation burden, or patterns of communication breakdown may all serve as indicators that system conditions are shifting.

When interpreted alongside frontline observations, these signals allow healthcare organizations to intervene before vulnerabilities escalate into patient harm. Rather than reacting to adverse events after they occur, leaders can examine early indicators that suggest increasing system stress and respond through targeted redesign efforts.

Recent research has highlighted both the promise and the risks associated with artificial intelligence in healthcare. Predictive algorithms may improve detection of clinical deterioration and operational risk, yet poorly integrated technologies can introduce new forms of complexity, bias, and workflow disruption [9–12]. Safe implementation therefore requires careful attention to how digital tools interact with clinical decision-making, care coordination, and the cognitive demands placed on frontline professionals.

The investigative methods discussed throughout this book were developed to help healthcare teams see and understand how complex care systems function in practice. Until recently, however, the ability to observe system behavior depended largely on direct human observation, retrospective investigation, and manual analysis of limited data. These approaches remain essential for understanding the realities of clinical work, yet they also impose practical limits on how much of a system can be observed at any given time.

Emerging digital capabilities are beginning to change these conditions. Advances in artificial intelligence, simulation, sensing, and digital modeling are creating new ways to observe, analyze, and redesign healthcare environments. These capabilities do not replace the investigative approaches described in previous chapters. Instead, they extend them. They allow healthcare organizations to examine system behavior at scales and levels of detail that were previously difficult to achieve through observation alone.

For patient safety professionals, these technologies introduce an important shift in perspective. The discipline of patient safety has traditionally focused on learning from adverse events and redesigning systems in response to identified failures. Digital modeling and artificial intelligence create the possibility of identifying patterns of system strain much earlier, testing potential redesigns before implementation, and monitoring care environments in ways that support continuous learning. Understanding these emerging capabilities is therefore not simply a matter of technological awareness. It is part of understanding how the work of patient safety may evolve in the coming decades.

## Digital Twins and Simulation for Safer System Design

Digital modeling technologies may allow healthcare organizations to construct detailed virtual representations of clinical systems. These models, often described as digital twins, are dynamic virtual representations of real systems that allow organizations to explore how changes in staffing, workflow design, technologies, or patient volume may influence system performance [13].

A digital twin functions as a continuously updated simulation of a real environment. Data drawn from operational systems, clinical workflows, and technology platforms can be used to recreate how a hospital unit, outpatient clinic, or diagnostic service operates in practice. Once constructed, these models allow leaders and improvement teams to test proposed interventions within simulated environments before implementing them in live clinical settings.

By modeling how changes in staffing patterns, patient acuity, or technology configuration affect system behavior, digital twins may allow organizations to identify unintended consequences earlier in the design process. A proposed workflow redesign, for example, could be simulated to examine how it influences clinician workload, communication patterns, patient throughput, or diagnostic delays. These simulations may reveal vulnerabilities that would otherwise become visible only after implementation in real clinical environments.

Such digital representations allow organizations to experiment with different configurations of staffing models, equipment placement, patient flow, and information systems. By observing how these variables interact within simulated environments, healthcare teams may be able to identify potential safety risks earlier in the design process. Rather than implementing changes and learning from failure, organizations may increasingly learn through simulation and experimentation before those changes affect real patients.

These developments align closely with the principles of design thinking discussed throughout this book. Design methods emphasize observing real-world behavior, generating alternative solutions, and testing those ideas iteratively before large-scale implementation. When combined with digital modeling, simulation, and human-centered design approaches, these methods may allow healthcare organizations to prototype safer systems more rapidly and explore multiple design possibilities before committing to a single approach.

Although these technologies remain in relatively early stages of development within healthcare, they illustrate the growing potential for digital tools to support anticipatory patient safety. Importantly, these technologies must remain embedded within human-centered systems of care. Their value lies not in replacing clinical judgment but in expanding visibility into the patterns that shape system performance and design.

## Artificial Intelligence and Continuous System Sensing

While digital twins are often used to simulate how proposed changes may influence system performance, artificial intelligence offers a related but distinct capability: the ability to analyze real-world data streams and detect emerging patterns of risk within complex healthcare systems.

Modern clinical environments generate enormous volumes of data through electronic health records, physiologic monitoring systems, operational platforms, and communication tools. Much of this information is stored but rarely analyzed in ways that reveal how system conditions evolve over time. Artificial intelligence systems are increasingly capable of analyzing large volumes of clinical and operational data to detect patterns that may be difficult for humans to identify through traditional analysis.

Predictive algorithms are already being used to detect early signs of patient deterioration, identify potential medication interactions, and flag operational risks such as delays in care transitions or abnormal documentation patterns. These tools expand the capacity of healthcare organizations to recognize emerging safety threats before they become visible through traditional reporting mechanisms.

Another emerging possibility is the use of artificial intelligence agents as continuous observers of complex healthcare systems. These agents are software systems capable of analyzing large volumes of data in real time to detect patterns across multiple sources simultaneously [10]. Instead of relying solely on voluntary reporting or retrospective analysis, intelligent systems could continuously analyze clinical documentation, communication networks, operational data, and physiologic monitoring streams. Subtle changes in workflow patterns, unusual medication ordering behavior, communication delays, or shifts in documentation activity may all serve as early indicators that system conditions are changing.

In such environments, patient safety surveillance may become more proactive and dynamic. Rather than relying primarily on episodic investigations triggered by adverse events, healthcare organizations may develop the capacity to observe patterns of system behavior as they emerge. Signals generated through operational data, clinical documentation, environmental sensing, and communication networks could allow organizations to detect subtle shifts in system conditions before those shifts produce visible harm.

In this model, patient safety begins to resemble a form of continuous system sensing. The work of patient safety professionals expands from investigating failures after they occur to interpreting the evolving signals that indicate how safe performance is being sustained or threatened within complex care environments.

## Governance and the Expanding Role of Patient Safety Teams

The integration of artificial intelligence into healthcare environments introduces new responsibilities for patient safety professionals. Algorithms may behave differently when applied to new populations, interact with clinical workflows in unexpected ways, or produce recommendations that clinicians interpret inconsistently. Ensuring that these systems function safely requires ongoing monitoring of model performance, evaluation of unintended consequences, and collaboration among clinicians, engineers, and data scientists.

Importantly, the presence of intelligent monitoring systems introduces new governance responsibilities for healthcare organizations. Mechanisms are needed to evaluate how these models function, how they influence clinical workflows, and whether their outputs are interpreted appropriately by clinicians and operational leaders. Patient safety teams may therefore become stewards not only of the algorithmic systems that increasingly shape clinical processes [10, 11].

This has implications for the discipline of patient safety itself. Traditionally, patient safety teams have focused primarily on investigating adverse events and implementing corrective actions. In increasingly digital healthcare environments, their responsibilities may expand to include interpreting signals generated by predictive analytics, participating in algorithm governance, and contributing to the design of safer clinical workflows.

This work may involve interpreting patterns identified through predictive analytics, collaborating with data scientists to understand model behavior, and participating in the design of systems that integrate human judgment with automated insights. Safety professionals may also contribute to the evaluation of digital tools before implementation and to the redesign of clinical environments so that technologies support safe performance under conditions of complexity.

In this sense, the discipline of patient safety may move closer to fields such as systems engineering, human factors, and design. Rather than focusing primarily on retrospective analysis of failure, patient safety professionals may increasingly shape how healthcare systems learn, adapt, and sustain safe performance over time.

## Reframing the Discipline

Advancing anticipatory patient safety requires more than new technologies or analytic tools. It also requires a shift in how healthcare professionals understand their role within complex clinical systems.

For generations, clinicians have been trained primarily as experts in diagnosis and treatment. Their professional identity centers on the knowledge and judgment required to care for individual patients. This focus remains essential. Yet modern healthcare increasingly reveals that patient outcomes are shaped by both clinical expertise and by the systems through which care is delivered.

## Participants in System Design

Clinical environments influence how information is perceived, how decisions are made, and how teams coordinate their work. Communication structures determine how quickly concerns are escalated. Technology interfaces shape how clinicians interpret patient data. Staffing models influence the cognitive demands placed on healthcare professionals during periods of high patient volume.

Recognizing these influences invites a broader understanding of professional responsibility. Clinicians remain caregivers, but they are also participants in complex systems whose design influences patient outcomes. When healthcare professionals learn to examine how workflows evolve, how technologies shape cognition, and how organizational structures influence coordination, they gain the ability to identify vulnerabilities that might otherwise remain hidden.

## Expanding Interdisciplinary Collaboration

Designing safer systems requires expertise that extends beyond clinical knowledge. Human factors specialists, engineers, designers, data scientists, and operational leaders each contribute perspectives that illuminate different aspects of system behavior.

When these disciplines collaborate with clinicians who understand the realities of patient care, healthcare organizations gain a more complete understanding of how safety emerges within complex environments. Interdisciplinary collaboration allows teams to examine problems from multiple perspectives and to develop solutions that account for both technical and human factors considerations.

## Safety as Shared Organizational Responsibility

Over time, this change transforms how healthcare organizations approach patient safety. Safety is no longer viewed solely as the responsibility of specialized departments or investigation teams. Instead, it becomes a shared commitment distributed across the organization.

Clinicians, leaders, designers, and technical specialists all contribute to the ongoing work of examining and refining the systems through which care is delivered. When organizations cultivate cultures that encourage curiosity, reflection, and interdisciplinary collaboration, they create conditions in which safety improvement becomes part of everyday clinical work rather than an activity confined to isolated improvement projects.

## Implications for the Future of Patient Safety

The perspective developed throughout this book suggests that the next stage of patient safety will depend less on identifying new categories of error and more on strengthening the ability of healthcare systems to observe, understand, and redesign their own behavior. As healthcare delivery becomes increasingly complex, organizations will require new capabilities for observing system performance, interpreting emerging signals of risk, and adapting care environments in response. Methods drawn from design thinking, human factors engineering, and systems science offer practical approaches for developing these capabilities within clinical settings.

These developments also have implications for research and policy. Patient safety scholarship has historically focused on the analysis of adverse events and the evaluation of targeted interventions. While this work remains essential, future research may increasingly examine how healthcare organizations develop the institutional capacity to observe system behavior and learn from everyday clinical work. Similarly, policy frameworks that emphasize transparency and accountability may gradually expand to support proactive system redesign and continuous organizational learning.

The ideas presented in this book also highlight the importance of interdisciplinary collaboration in advancing patient safety. Clinicians, designers, engineers, human factors specialists, and data scientists each bring perspectives that illuminate different aspects of system behavior. When these disciplines work together, healthcare organizations gain the ability to examine complex environments with greater clarity and to design systems that better support safe care under real-world conditions.

Looking ahead, it is reasonable to imagine that a patient safety department ten years from now may look quite different from many departments today. In addition to investigating adverse events and supporting improvement initiatives, patient safety teams may help evaluate digital tools before implementation, monitor the performance and consequences of predictive models, interpret system-level signals of strain, and collaborate with engineers, designers, and data scientists to test new care models. In such environments, patient safety professionals may spend less of their time looking only backward at harm and more of their time helping organizations understand how complex systems behave, how those systems can be redesigned, and how safe performance can be sustained as care delivery and technology continue to evolve.

## Designing the Conditions for Safer Care

The history of patient safety has been shaped by the careful study of harm. Investigations into medical error revealed that failures in healthcare rarely arise from a single mistake or isolated lapse in judgment. Instead, they emerge from the interaction of people, technologies, workflows, and environments operating under conditions of complexity and constraint.

Recognizing this reality transformed how healthcare understands safety. Responsibility expanded beyond individual clinicians to include the systems in which care is delivered. Yet acknowledging that safety is systemic represents only the first step. The deeper challenge lies in developing the capacity to design systems that support safe care under the unpredictable conditions of clinical practice.

Throughout this book, design thinking has been presented as a disciplined approach for examining and improving complex systems. Methods such as contextual observation, journey mapping, service blueprinting, and structured validation allow healthcare organizations to see how care actually unfolds rather than how it is assumed to occur. Measurement frameworks allow teams to evaluate whether redesign efforts improve reliability and reduce system strain. Governance structures, workforce capability, and institutional learning mechanisms ensure that insights generated through local redesign efforts inform broader organizational decision-making.

Looking ahead, the tools available to support anticipatory safety will continue to expand. Advances in sensing technologies, artificial intelligence, and digital modeling may allow healthcare systems to detect subtle patterns of risk that were previously invisible. Yet the future of patient safety will depend less on any single technological breakthrough than on the collective ability of healthcare organizations to design systems that learn. Organizations capable of observing how care unfolds, interpreting emerging signals of strain, and redesigning systems in response will be better prepared to navigate the complexity that defines modern healthcare.

## Conclusion

The history of patient safety has shown with increasing clarity that harm rarely arises from isolated mistakes alone. It emerges through the interaction of people, technologies, workflows, environments, and organizational conditions that together shape what safe performance requires and how difficult that performance becomes to sustain. Recognizing this changed the field. It redirected attention from individual blame toward the systems in which care is delivered. That reorientation, however, does not complete the work. It only establishes where the next set of responsibilities begins.

What follows from that recognition is more demanding than better retrospective analysis alone. If harm is produced through the ordinary design and operation of care systems, then patient safety cannot remain primarily a discipline of explanation after failure. It must also become a discipline of earlier recognition, deliberate testing, and redesign under real conditions. The methods developed throughout this book matter because they make it possible to study how care is actually carried out, where strain gathers, and which assumptions no longer hold before visible failure becomes the main source of evidence.

That shift carries institutional implications. Healthcare organizations will need to do more than investigate adverse events competently. They will need to build the capacity to notice weak signals, to examine how work is being sustained through adaptation, to test change before it is embedded at scale, and to treat design itself as a matter of safety governance. In that environment, patient safety becomes less episodic and more continuous. It becomes less dependent on breakdown as the first condition for learning. It also becomes more closely tied to leadership, operational design, digital infrastructure, workforce conditions, and the everyday realities through which care is delivered.

None of this makes patient safety simpler. It makes its demands harder to ignore. The systems of modern healthcare are not becoming less complex, less technological, or less interdependent. They are becoming more so. In such settings, it is no longer enough to ask whether organizations learn from failure when failure becomes undeniable. A more difficult question now stands in front of the field: whether healthcare is willing to redesign the conditions that make harm more likely while those conditions are still taking shape. Much of the future of patient safety may depend on how seriously that question is taken.

# References


1. Institute of Medicine. To err is human: building a safer health system. Washington, DC: National Academies Press; 2000.
2. Reason J. Human error. Cambridge: Cambridge University Press; 1990.
3. Hollnagel E. Safety-I and safety-II: the past and future of safety management. Farnham: Ashgate Publishing; 2014.
4. Hollnagel E, Braithwaite J, Wears RL, editors. Resilient health care. Farnham: Ashgate Publishing; 2013.
5. Braithwaite J, Wears RL, Hollnagel E. Resilient health care: turning patient safety on its head. Int J Qual Health Care. 2015;27(5):418–20. https://doi.org/10.1093/intqhc/mzv063.
6. World Health Organization. Global Patient Safety Action Plan 2021–2030: towards eliminating avoidable harm in health care. Geneva: World Health Organization; 2021.
7. Carayon P, Schoofs Hundt A, Karsh BT, Gurses AP, Alvarado CJ, Smith M, Brennan PF. Work system design for patient safety: the SEIPS model. Qual Saf Health Care. 2006;15(Suppl 1):i50–8. https://doi.org/10.1136/qshc.2005.015842.
8. Awad S, Begg R, Loveday T, Baysari MT. Using human centred design and human factors to support a rapid health information technology patient safety response. BMC Health Serv Res. 2025;25(1):1143. https://doi.org/10.1186/s12913-025-13293-5.
9. Topol EJ. Deep medicine: how artificial intelligence can make healthcare human again. New York: Basic Books; 2019.
10. Sendak MP, D'Arcy J, Kashyap S, Gao M, Nichols M, Corey K, Ratliff W, Balu S. A path for translation of machine learning products into healthcare delivery. EMJ Innov. 2020;4(1):1–8. https://doi.org/10.33590/emjinnov/19-00172.
11. Rajkomar A, Dean J, Kohane I. Machine learning in medicine. N Engl J Med. 2019;380(14):1347–58. https://doi.org/10.1056/NEJMra1814259.
12. Topol EJ. High-performance medicine: the convergence of human and artificial intelligence. Nat Med. 2019;25(1):44–56. https://doi.org/10.1038/s41591-018-0300-7.
13. Jones D, Snider C, Nassehi A, Yon J, Hicks B. Characterising the digital twin: a systematic literature review. CIRP J Manuf Sci Technol. 2020;29:36–52. https://doi.org/10.1016/j.cirpj.2020.02.002.

# Index




K. Rasmussen, *Rethinking Patient Safety*,
https://doi.org/10.1007/978-3-032-26054-3

**D**

## U



## V



## W

GPSR Compliance

*The European Union's (EU) General Product Safety Regulation (GPSR) is a set of rules that requires consumer products to be safe and our obligations to ensure this.*

*If you have any concerns about our products, you can contact us on ProductSafety@springernature.com*

In case Publisher is established outside the EU, the EU authorized representative is:

Springer Nature Customer Service Center GmbH
Europaplatz 3
69115 Heidelberg, Germany

**Batch number: 10755079**

Printed by Printforce, the Netherlands